Clinical Teaching Made Easy

WB18
MCK

Note
Health care practice and knowledge are constantly changing and developing as new research and treatments, changes in procedures, drugs and equipment become available.
The author and publishers have, as far as is possible, taken care to confirm that the information complies with the latest standards of practice and legislation.

Clinical Teaching Made Easy

A practical guide to teaching and learning in clinical settings

Judy McKimm and Tim Swanwick

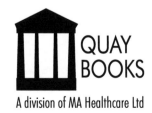

QUAY
BOOKS

A division of MA Healthcare Ltd

Quay Books Division, MA Healthcare Ltd, St Jude's Church, Dulwich Road, London
SE24 0PB

British Library Cataloguing-in-Publication Data
A catalogue record is available for this book

© MA Healthcare Limited 2010
ISBN-10: 1 85642 408 1; ISBN-13: 978 1 85642 408 0

Printed by CLE, Huntingdon, Cambridgeshire

Contents

About the editors   vi
Contributors   vii
Acknowledgements   ix
Preface   viii

CHAPTERS

1	Introduction	1
2	Assessing learning needs	7
3	Setting learning objectives	17
4	Curriculum and course design	29
5	Giving effective feedback	41
6	Supervision	51
7	Facilitating learning in the workplace	61
8	Improve your lecturing	69
9	Small group teaching	79
10	Involving patients in clinical teaching	91
11	Workplace-based assessment	103
12	Interprofessional learning	113
13	e-learning for clinical teachers	123
14	Using simulation in clinical education	133
15	Structured assessments of clinical competence	145
16	Appraisal	153
17	Careers support	163
18	Mentoring	173
19	Managing poor performance	185
20	Diversity, equal opportunities and human rights	195
21	Introduction to educational research	207
22	Professional development of medical educators	219
23	Assuring and enhancing educational quality	231
	Index	241

About the editors

Judy McKimm, MBA BA (Hons) Cert Ed SFHEA FAcadMed is Dean and Professor of Medical Education, Swansea University. Judy has extensive international curriculum development, teaching and research experience in undergraduate and postgraduate medical, health professions and social care education, in faculty development and in educational and clinical leadership development. Judy publishes widely, holds a number of editorial positions, is a Visiting Professor at the University of Bedfordshire and was previously Pro Dean (Health and Social Practice) Unitec New Zealand.

Professor Tim Swanwick, MA MBBS DRCOG DCH FRCGP MA (Ed) FAcadMed is Dean of Professional Development in the London Deanery where he has an extensive portfolio that includes faculty development, coaching and mentoring, careers and clinical leadership. Tim has a broad experience in postgraduate medical education, has written and researched widely and holds a number of other appointments including Visiting Professor at the University of Bedfordshire, Visiting Fellow at the Institute of Education of London University and Honorary Senior Lecturer at Imperial College.

Contributors

Dr Mark Barrow, MSc, EdD, DipTchg, Associate Dean (Education), Faculty of Medical and Health Sciences, University of Auckland, Auckland, New Zealand.

Dr Katharine Boursicot, BSc (Hons) MBMS, MRCOG, MAHPE, Reader in Medical Education, Head of Assessment, St George's, University of London, London, UK.

Dr Howard Borkett-Jones, MB BS,FRCS,FCEM,MA(Med Ed); Consultant in Emergency Medicine, and Associate Medical Director for Education and Training, Watford General Hospital, Watford, Hertfordshire.

Dulcie Jane Brake, MEd, BA (Ed), PGDipEd, Academic Literacy Adviser, Faculty of Social and Health Sciences, Unitec New Zealand, Auckland, New Zealand.

Dr Iain Doherty, PhD, MLitt, BA (Hons), Director, Learning Technology Unit, Faculty of Medical Health Sciences, University of Auckland, New Zealand.

Dr Nav Chana, MA, FRCGP, MB. BS, Associate Director Postgraduate GP Education, London Deanery, Honorary Senior Lecturer, St George's.

Dr Caroline Elton, BA(Hons), PGCE, Ph.D, C.Psychol, Head of Careers Advice and Planning, London Deanery, London, UK.

Dr Kirsty Forrest, MBChB, BSc (Hons), MMEd, PGDip Anaes, FRCA, FAcadMed, Honorary Clinical Senior Lecturer and Consultant Anaesthetist, Academic Unit of Anaesthesia, University of Leeds, Leeds and Clinical Education Advisor, Yorkshire and Humber Deanery.

Dr Helen Halpern, MB BS, FRCGP, MSysPsych, GP Tutor and Course Tutor in Supervision Skills, London Deanery, London, UK.

Sam Held, MA, PGCert (Higher Education Leadership), Patient and Family Services Manager, North Shore Hospice, Auckland, New Zealand.

Clare Morris, MA (Ed), BSc (Hons), FHEA, Associate Dean. Postgraduate Medical School, University of Bedfordshire, Luton, UK.

Doug Parkin BA (Hons), MInstLM, FHEA, AssocCIPD, Head of Staff and Educational Development, London School of Hygiene and Tropical Medicine, University of London, UK.

Dr Rebecca Viney, MBBS, FHEA, Cert (ed), Dip AD, Dip Occ Med, Coaching and Mentoring Lead and Associate Director Postgraduate GP education, London Deanery, London, UK and General Practitioner, London, UK.

Helen Webb, BA (Hons), MCIPD, Training and Consulting Manager, Equality Works Ltd, London, UK.

Acknowledgements

We would like to express our gratitude to our co-authors for their thoughtful contributions to the book, together with those colleagues, students and trainees who have helped to shape our views and practice of clinical learning and teaching. Thanks also to Sam Hobbs and Jon Wilkinson for helping to bring this project to fruition and to Professor Shelley Heard, whose idea it is was in the first place.

Preface

In 2007, the London Deanery, an organisation responsible for the postgraduate training of over 12 500 doctors and dentists, embarked on an ambitious programme of faculty development. One of the outputs of that programme was a series of e-learning modules to aid the professional development of London's own postgraduate training network across a large number of Acute, Foundation Primary Care and Mental Health Trusts. The modules, condensed and supplemented with new material, were subsequently published as a monthly series of articles in the *British Journal of Hospital Medicine* and are collated here in *Clinical Teaching Made Easy: A practical guide to teaching and learning in clinical settings*.

This is a practical book. Chapters have been written for the clinician, rather than the academic educator, and our intention is to provide comprehensive coverage of all aspects of clinical teaching and training of immediate relevance to the health service setting. If, after reading a given chapter, you want to explore a particular topic further then we recommend that you visit www.londondeanery.ac.uk/facultydevelopment where you can find the full suite of open access e-learning modules complete with a range of supporting material.

Although *Clinical Teaching Made Easy: A practical guide to teaching and learning in a clinical setting* was written with the medic in mind, where possible we have tried to pull out generic themes and highlight multiprofessional messages. Many topics – patient involvement, workplace-based assessment, supervision etc – have no uniprofessional ownership and readily translate across a range of clinical contexts. We therefore invite colleagues from all healthcare professions where learning and teaching takes place in the clinical setting, to join us in this exploration of what it means to be an effective clinical teacher.

Judy McKimm and Tim Swanwick
August 2010

CHAPTER I

Introduction

Tim Swanwick

At the time when this chapter first appeared in the *British Journal of Hospital Medicine*, postgraduate medical education had just emerged from the rather prolonged and difficult labour of *Modernising Medical Careers*, a wide-reaching programme of educational reform. Having restructured, and to a certain extent formalised, postgraduate medical education, the next task for both government and the regulator was to improve its quality. Many other professions, such as nursing, already had a long and enviable track record of high quality service-based education, and medicine clearly had some catching up to do. One of the hardest tasks was to dispel the belief that clinical teaching and training was something that could be fitted in and around the service-day, requiring no special ability or skills on the part of the clinical teacher. This chapter then lays out that (long over-due) challenge to medical teachers, namely that engaging in faculty development, or teaching the teachers programmes, should be an essential requirement for educational practice, no longer an optional extra. We apologise to colleagues from other disciplines for the uniprofessional nature of what follows, who we recommend skip the next few pages and go straight on to the 'business' of clinical teaching presented in the rest of the book. In the meantime, doctors, read on.

In a quiet and not often visited corner of the General Medical Council's Good Medical Practice (2001) - paragraphs 15 and 16 if you're interested - lie two important statements. Firstly that:

> *Teaching, training, appraising and assessing doctors and students are important for the care of patients now and in the future. You should be willing to contribute to these activities.*

A willingness to be involved in clinical teaching then is a professional responsibility. But the GMC doesn't stop there, insisting that:

> *If you are involved in teaching you must develop the skills, attitudes and practices of a competent teacher.*

What this means is that it is that all doctors with clinical teaching or training responsibilities have a duty to undertake some form of educational training and development. With the introduction of revalidation, implicit in the GMC's statement is that doctors who train will need to provide evidence that they have attained the appropriate skills, attitudes and competences. Universities arrived at this point some time ago after the Dearing Report (1997) called for improvements to the quality of teaching in Higher Education. National standards are now embedded in the accreditation processes of the Higher Education Academy (accessed Jan 2009). Similar requirements are echoed in Tomorrow's Doctors (General Medical Council 2003), the GMC's framework of guidance for UK medical schools, which demands that clinical teachers should participate in staff-development programmes.

Regulation in postgraduate medical education is catching up and with the establishment of the Postgraduate Medical Education and Training Board (PMETB) in 2005 (a short-lived organisation as it happens, now subsumed within the GMC) a raft of 'standards' documents have appeared. The emphasis here is on supervision rather than teaching, but the tenor is the same and the GMC (PMETB)'s over-arching Generic Standards for Training (Postgraduate Medical Education and Training Board 2008) requires that consultant trainers with a supervisory responsibility are both selected for their role and can demonstrate their ability.

Finally, driven by the recognition that the quality of medical teaching and training is inextricably linked to the quality of patient care, is the Department of Health's policy document, A High Quality Workforce: NHS Next Stage Review (Department of Health 2008). Lord Darzi's paper published last year outlines the government's intention that all educational supervisors in secondary care undergo 'mandatory training and performance review as currently exists in primary care'.

So there you have it. Undertaking a 'teaching the teachers' programme is to be a mandatory requirement whether you teach undergraduates or supervise foundation doctors or specialty trainees. And most consultant teachers will have contact with learners at all three stages of training.

So what are the skills, attitudes and practices of a competent teacher?

Medical education is a hybrid discipline that has appropriated both theory and practice from other areas of mainstream education. However, it has also made some significant contributions to the field, such as in the areas of problem based learning, simulation and assessment and in its practice, medical education has a number of features that set it apart from other educational disciplines.

In medical schools, these unique features are most notable outside the lecture theatre, an efficient but perhaps ineffective vehicle for mass knowledge-delivery that we continue to share with higher education. Undergraduate medical education now makes extensive and creative use of a variety of teaching methods including skills labs, e-learning and small group discussion. The rise of integrated and problem-based curricula exposes students to a wide variety of clinical areas from early in their medical training and the tyranny of final year examinations has given way to more authentic assessments such as objective structure clinical examinations (Boursicot et al 2007) and portfolios (Driessen et al 2003) delivered across, and integrated with, the course.

Postgraduate medical education is also changing, albeit slowly. Historically training at this level has been loosely structured on an apprenticeship model where learning through observation, modelling and graded participation occurred in an idiosyncratic and haphazard fashion, supported by often serendipitous access to formal educational events such as grand rounds, half-day release courses and departmental meetings. With the reduction of hours brought about by the New Deal and the European Working Time Directive (Department of Health 2004, Pickersgill 2001), and an increased public and professional accountability, there has been widespread recognition that 'learning by lurking' is not enough to guarantee the production of safe and competent clinicians. From the Calman reforms of the 1990s onwards (Paice et al 2000), postgraduate medical education and training has undergone a slow but inexorable transformation.

The new training places a strong emphasis on supervision, both with an eye to patient safety but the also the oversight of professional development of trainees (Kilminster et al 2007). Trainers in all specialties are expected to deliver against clearly defined competency-based curricula and work with a raft of centrally imposed workplace-based assessments. Formal learning opportunities are combined with work-based experience to deliver curricula and there is an increasing use of simulation and technology to promote the development of technical skills and non-technical skills.

So the competent clinical teacher may require a range of abilities from presenting lectures to facilitating small groups; from conducting developmental conversations to delivering formal workplace assessments; from offering feedback on a ward-based clinical examination to debriefing a full immersion team-based simulation.

Organisations and researchers and have attempted to capture the complexities of medical education in a number of competency frameworks (Wall and McAleer 2000, Hesketh 2001, London Deanery 2008). The most recent contributor is the UK's Academy of Medical Educators, an organisation whose expressed intent is to 'improve patient care through promoting excellence in medical teaching and learning' (Bligh and Brice, 2007). To achieve this, the Academy aims to provide a recognised framework in order that medical educators can demonstrate their expertise and achievements through accreditation against an agreed national standard. The Academy is also helping to develop a transparent career structure for specialist medical educators. But the Academy is just one example of what is an international trend. The 'professionalization' of clinical teaching can only continue to gather momentum. Politicians, the public and our professional bodies will require nothing less.

References

Bligh J, Brice J (2007) The Academy of Medical Educators: a professional home for medical educators in the UK. Medical Education **41**(7): 625-7.

Boursicot KAM, Roberts T and Burdick WP (2007) Structured assessments of clinical competence. In: Swanwick T, ed. Understanding Medical Education. Association for the Study of Medical Education, Edinburgh.

Darzi A (2008) A High Quality Workforce: NHS Next Stage Review. Department of Health, London.

Department of Health (2004) European Working Time Directive (cited 2009 January 26th) Available from: http://www.dh.gov.uk/PolicyAndGuidance/ HumanResourcesAndTraining/WorkingDifferently/EuropeanWorkingTimeDirective

Dearing R (1999) Higher Education in the Learning Society: National Committee of Inquiry into Higher Education. HMSO, London.

Driessen EW et al (2003) Use of portfolios in early undergraduate medical training. Medical Teacher, 2003. **25**(1): 14-19.

General Medical Council (2001) Good Medical Practice. General Medical Council, London.

General Medical Council (2003) Tomorrow's Doctors. General Medical Council, London.

Hesketh EA et al (2001) A framework for developing excellence as a clinical educator. *Medical Education* **35**: 555-64.

Higher Education Academy (2009) The UK Professional Standards Framework for teaching and supporting learning in higher education. (cited 2009 January 26th); Available from: http://www.heacademy.ac.uk/ourwork/professional/recognition.

London Deanery (2008) Faculty Development: A Curriculum for Clinical Teachers. (cited 2009 January 26th); Available from: http://www.faculty.londondeanery.ac.uk/ curriculum-for-clinical-teachers.

Kilminster S et al (2007) AMEE Guide #27 Effective educational and clinical supervision *Medical Teacher* **29**: 2-19

Paice E et al (2000) Trainee satisfaction before and after the Calman reforms of specialist training: questionnaire survey *British Medical Journal* **320**(7238): 832-836.

Pickersgill, T (2001) The European working time directive for doctors in training. *British Medical Journal* **323**(7324):1266

Postgraduate Medical Education and Training Board (2008) Generic Standards for Training. Postgraduate Medical Education and Training Board, London.

Wall D and McAleer S (2000) Teaching the consultant teachers: identifying the core content. *Medical Education* **34**(2):131-138.

CHAPTER 2

Assessing learning needs

Judy McKimm and Tim Swanwick

Clinical teachers and educational supervisors work with a range of students and trainees on different programmes. Learners from diverse backgrounds have different learning needs which can be difficult to assess. Teachers who pay attention to individual learners' needs will help learners get the most from their training. This can be enhanced through the use of tools such as professional development plans and formal assessments.

This chapter explores the role of the clinical teacher in assessing the learning needs of students or trainees in the context of organizational and professional requirements. It considers how teachers can support individual students or trainees in formal and informal teaching situations and as part of their continuing personal and professional development and discusses some of the tools and techniques used for assessing learning needs.

The role of the clinical teacher

The role of a clinical teacher is complex. Teaching activities are often combined with clinical commitments and you may work with learners at different levels and with different professional requirements. Harden and Crosby (2000) define twelve different teaching roles (*Table 2.1*).

One of the main tasks of a clinical teacher is to support students or trainees in their professional development. This includes helping students and trainees to acquire clinical knowledge and skills, facilitating the development of appropriate professional attitudes and fostering self-directed, lifelong learning. One way of thinking about one's role in relation to learners is to think in terms of the trainees' or students' 'learning journey'. Planning the journey and assessing learning needs is an essential part of the journey.

In medicine, learners are working towards a professional qualification therefore their formal learning outcomes are already defined, typically as

Table 2.1. The twelve roles of the clinical teacher

Roles that require more educational expertise	Examiner	Planning or participating in formal examinations of students
		Curriculum evaluator
	Planner	Curriculum planner
		Course organizer
	Resource developer	Production of study guides
		Developing resource materials in the form of computer programmes, video or print
Roles that require more content expertise or knowledge	Information provider	Lecturer in classroom setting
		Teacher in practical or clinical setting
	Role model	On-the-job role model
		Role model in the teaching setting
	Facilitator	Mentor, personal adviser or tutor
		Learning facilitator

adapted from Harden and Crosby (2000)

a written curriculum, syllabus or programme of study which is assessed according to stated criteria. Each teaching or learning event needs to be relevant to the overall programme. Making oneself familiar with the intended or expected learning outcomes is a vital first step in assessing learning needs and planning teaching and learning activities.

Because learners' past experiences, learning styles, abilities and expectations vary, so do individual learning needs. Learning needs can be assessed formally and informally in teaching situations: the classroom, at the bedside or in the consulting room. Spencer (2003) suggests that teachers can optimize teaching and learning opportunities that arise in daily practice through planning, using appropriate questioning techniques and teaching in different clinical contexts. Clinical teachers also provide support, guidance and supervision for learners in their professional and personal development, appraisal and career advice.

Table 2.2. The Johari window		
	Known to self	**Unknown to self**
Known to others	Open	Blind
Known to self	Hidden	Unknown

What are we trying to achieve?

The attentive clinical teacher can support professional development in a number of ways, including through providing appropriate feedback (See Chapter 5). How this is done depends on the extent to which both teacher and student, or trainer and trainee are aware of the learner's strengths and weaknesses. The Johari window (Luft and Ingham, 1955) is a widely-used model that neatly summarizes these states of self-knowledge (*Table 2.2*).

The window is a two-by-two taxonomy of learning or development needs with the underlying assumption that if gaps or deficiencies are out in the open, then they can be more effectively addressed. The aim is to try to move learning needs into the 'open' quadrant where what needs to be learned is known both to the learner and to the teacher.

Where others can see his/her deficiencies or gaps but the learner cannot, the learner is said to be 'blind'. This is where the use of formative workplace-based assessments and a trusting relationship can help the learner become aware of his/her learning needs. Here, the teacher needs to help the learner learn something about him-/herself that he/she does not already know.

Where the learner is aware of his/her gaps or deficiencies but others are not, learning needs are said to be 'hidden'. Moving these into the open quadrant requires a high level of trust between the teacher and the learner so that learners feel able to admit weaknesses and deficiencies or reveal fears.

The 'unknown' quadrant represents those learning needs that are neither known to the teacher nor to the learner. This is where both teacher and learner need to work together to identify areas for further exploration. Multisource feedback and formal assessments have a role here in flagging up previously unidentified problem areas.

Another way of looking at these issues is the 'competency model' of professional development (Proctor, 2001; Hill, 2007) (*Table 2.3*). In this model teachers also help learners move through four stages of development: from unconscious incompetence, where the unskilled learner is also unaware of his/her failings, to unconscious competence, or a state of more intuitive or free-flowing expertise.

Table 2.3. Role of clinical teacher in supporting the development of professional competence

	Unconscious incompetence	Conscious inwcompetence	Conscious competence	Unconscious competence
Learner	Low level of competence. Unaware of failings	Low level of competence. Aware of failings but not having full skills to correct	Demonstrates competence but skills not fully internalised or integrated. Has to think about activities	Carries out tasks without thought. Skills internalised and routine. Little or no conscious awareness of detailed processes involved in activities
Clinical teacher: assessing learning or educational needs	Supportively helps learner to recognize weaknesses, identify any areas for development and become aware of learning/ development needs and thus conscious of 'incompetence'	Uses range of skills and techniques to assess learners' development in relation to defined expectations for the level and stage of learning. helps learner to develop and refine self-assessment skills. Reassures and supports	Helps learner to develop and refine skills, reinforces good practice and competence through positive regular feedback and a focus on areas for development and refinement of skills, additional knowledge required and an integration of competencies	Raise awareness of detail and unpacks processes for more advanced learning. Helps learner to identify areas of weakness/ bad habits that they may not be aware of

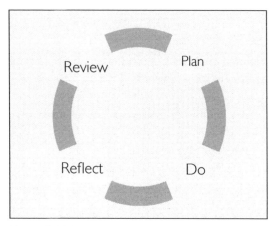

Figure 2.1. The plan, do, reflect, review cycle.

When and where to assess?

Identifying and assessing learning needs can be conceived as a part of the Kolb experiential learning cycle (Kolb, 1984) where the next steps on the learning journey arise from reflection on past experiences.

In practical terms, learning needs should be assessed at a number of points: at the start of a programme, meeting or teaching session, during the course of a programme or session to review progress, and at the end of a session or course of study to plan ongoing learning according to where learners are going next.

Before starting any teaching episode, the teacher needs to establish an understanding of where the learner is, the level he/she has reached, his/her past experience and his/her personal goals. As part of the overall planning process for a teaching session, the teacher will also have defined his/her aims of the session, the learning outcomes or objectives and possibly an assessment. At the start of the session, these should be explained to the learner to set the context for the learning and align the stated, formal learning outcomes with individual learners' educational needs. So how can this be done in busy clinical sessions?

Assessing learning needs can be done relatively informally and briefly at the start of a teaching session, simply by asking the learners what they would like to or what they expect to get out of the teaching session: a quick 'checking in'. Making this a routine part of any teaching session helps to avoid situations where the teacher is gamely plodding on regardless even though the learners are clearly disengaged with the process. During and towards the end of a teaching session, one needs to review how well the learners are achieving their learning goals, where they may have gone off track and what further learning or practice may be required. Keeping an eye on both the tasks that one wants learners to achieve as well as the process of learning will help to ensure that learning needs are met. If we go back to the learning journey, the journey (process) will be very different if you are flying, travelling by car or by boat; if you travel alone or in a group; if you are all setting off from the same place or if you are being led by a guide who is very familiar with where you want to go and has a good route map to hand.

Who assesses?

Assessing learning needs in teaching situations should then be a shared endeavour. Teachers play a key role in helping learners develop critical self-reflection and independence by providing opportunities for self-assessment of their clinical competence, knowledge, understanding and attitudes and by pointing out where there is a mismatch between self perception and observed behaviours. Building in simple questions such as 'how do you think that went...?' opens up opportunities for learners to routinely reflect on and review their performance.

One advantage of teacher assessment of learning needs is that experienced teachers know the programme and expected performance at different stages of practice. Highly competent teachers (Sadler, 1989) are knowledgeable, able to empathize with learners, are reflective about their own and others' skills and want to see learners improve and develop. However, different teachers' skills, experience or expertise can be variable, which is where standardized tools or techniques can help both teachers and learners.

Tools and techniques for assessing educational needs

Formal assessments assess learning at regular points against defined criteria. Well-designed assessments provide information for learners to help them identify where their learning has been effective and where they need to improve. Teachers can also use assessment results as one of the means to measure learners' progress and identify and agree learning needs. This section summarizes some instruments commonly used in clinical teaching and personal and professional development to assess learning or educational needs.

Professional 'conversations'

> *'Even for established professionals, groups learn together through an often asymmetric co-participation in practice. Clinical practice is littered with tales told in conversations about difficulties and disasters... which can lead to reconsideration of practice, reflection and adaptive learning by the wider audience' (Pitts, 2007).*

The professional conversation is being increasingly formalized in medical education, e.g. through case-based discussion, and is used as a stimulus for ongoing professional development. It aligns with reflective practice, enabling both 'reflection in action' and 'reflection on action' (Schön, 1983; Launer, 2002).

By encouraging story-telling, narrative and conversation in a structured way, the teacher can work with the learner to help him/her identify significant elements, learning points and areas for further reflection or development. Care must be taken to avoid the conversation turning into a chat between friends, a paternalistic debate or an opportunity for unfounded criticism. Defining a 'learning contract' (Solomon, 1992) in terms of agreeing outcomes, a structure, prompt questions and timeframe helps to set clear boundaries around the conversation. One specific way of structuring a professional conversation is around a significant or critical incident.

Significant event analysis

> *'The structured and deliberate review of significant events has been advocated as a useful way to encourage reflection' (Brookfield, 1990).*

Significant event analysis can help learners make sense of events that, for one reason or another, evoke an emotional response, cause them to take stock, expose a gap in understanding or capabilities or cause them to think differently. The event need not cause anxiety or distress, it can be positive. This is a useful tool that you might use as a trigger to identify learning needs, or to reflect more deeply about an issue or situation. A common framework is:

- The learner or other member of the team raises an event as significant
- Each learner describes their event in their own way without interruptions (what happened)
- The teacher asks each learner to identify his/her initial thoughts and feelings (how did you feel about it?)
- Then follows an analysis or evaluation of the event (why do you think it happened this way or what do you think was going on?)
- Conclusions and implications for learning and development are drawn (what do you take forward from this? what do you think you've learned from this?)
- The significant event is usually then written up and filed in a learning log or personal development plan.

The key features of successful significant event analysis are that it should be a positive experience for all involved, it should result in some improvement in patient care and it is about development – not blame. Significant event sessions must be handled with sensitivity and care with enough time for debriefing (Henderson et al, 2002).

Formal assessments tools

Learning needs lurking in the blind or unknown quadrants of the Johari window can be surfaced through the use of formal assessment tools. These may be knowledge-based tests such as the multiple choice progress tests used in undergraduate medicine, objective structured assessments of clinical competence or one of the ever-increasing number of workplace-based assessments which have found favour in postgraduate medical education such as the mini-clinical evaluation exercise or direct observation of procedural skills.

Audit

Audit compares actual performance against a set of criteria and standards. It is therefore a powerful tool for learning as it reports the outcomes of what we actually do. Conducting small-scale audits of actual performance is a useful vehicle for identifying areas for future development and is usually a requirement of both undergraduate and postgraduate training programmes.

Personal development plans

These are formal means by which an individual (normally working with a teacher, mentor or supervisor) sets out the goals, strategies and intended outcomes of learning and training. These are typically developed in alignment with professional programmes of study or to meet requirements from regulatory or statutory bodies around continuing professional development and revalidation to retain a licence to practice, stay on a professional register and demonstrate professional standing.

A well-structured plan should clearly define timeframes, activities and outcomes to meet the defined goals and specify dates for review and meetings with teachers, supervisors or line managers. Plans will vary between individuals. Learning activities may include formal and informal training, reading, attending meetings, observing colleagues, practising clinical skills, refreshing or learning new study skills or developing new skills to meet a career goal (Jennings, 2007).

Portfolios

Portfolios pull together 'evidence' and information from a range of sources to demonstrate continuing professional development. Students, trainees and established practitioners are all increasingly required to a learning portfolio. In some medical schools and training programmes portfolios may also form part of the assessment process. Evidence collected is commonly linked together by a reflective diary, commentary or account of development over a specified timeframe enabling the reader to 'make sense' of the portfolio in terms of the individual's professional development and context.

Portfolios may be written or electronic in form and many have formal roles in appraisal and accreditation or review processes. They typically include a personal development plan, appraisal records (including academic appraisals, 360° appraisals, multisource feedback forms from patients, colleagues and others), research papers or other publications, conference papers, critical or significant incident analysis, attendance certificates from training events, clinical meetings, conferences, assessment results from training courses and other evidence requirements.

Conclusions

Assessing the learning needs of students and trainees is an activity that clinical teachers carry out on a day-to-day basis, both formally and informally and in a range of contexts. It is an essential element of effective teaching and supervision and is becoming increasingly more formalized as part of continuing professional development.

KEY POINTS

- Assessing learning needs is a key role of the clinical teacher in supporting learning and professional development.
- Programme learning outcomes, feedback from assessments and individual learning 'wants' all contribute towards defining current learning needs.
- It is important to build in time for assessing learning needs and checking they have been met.
- Assessment of learning needs can be carried out informally through professional conversations.
- Structured tools for assessing learning needs include significant event analysis, formal assessment instruments, audit, professional development plans and portfolios.

References

Brookfield S (1990) Using critical incidents to explore learners' assumptions. In: Mezirow J, ed. *Fostering Critical Reflection in Adulthood*. Jossey Bass, San Francisco: 177–93

Harden RM, Crosby JR (2000) *The good teacher is more than a lecturer: The twelve roles of the teacher*. AMEE Education Guide No 20, AMEE, Dundee: 124

Henderson E, Berlin A, Freeman G, Fuller J (2002) Twelve tips for promoting significant incident analysis to enhance reflection in undergraduate medical students. *Med Teach* **24**(2): 121–4

Hill F (2007) Feedback to enhance student learning: Facilitating interactive feedback on clinical skills. *International Journal of Clinical Skills* **1**(1): 21–4

Kolb DA (1984) *Experiential learning: Experience as the source of learning and development*. Prentice Hall, Englewood-Cliffs, NJ

Jennings SF (2007) Personal development plans and self-directed learning for healthcare professionals: are they evidence based? *Postgrad Med J* **83**: 518–24

Launer J (2002) *Narrative Based Primary Care: a practical guide*. Radcliffe Medical Press, Abingdon

Luft J, Ingham H (1955) The Johari window, a graphic model of interpersonal awareness. *Proceedings of the western training laboratory in group development*. UCLA, Los Angeles

Pitts J (2007) *Portfolios, Personal Development and Reflective Practice*. ASME UME series, ASME, Edinburgh: 14

Proctor B (2001) Training for supervision attitude, skills and intention. In: Cutcliffe J, Butterworth T, Proctor B, eds. *Fundamental Themes in Clinical Supervision*. Routledge, London

Sadler DR (1989) Formative assessment and the design of instructional systems. *Instructional Science* **18**: 119–44

Schön D (1983) *The Reflective Practitioner. How professionals think in action*. Temple Smith, London

Spencer J (2003) BMJ ABC of Learning and Teaching in Medicine: Learning and teaching in the clinical environment. *BMJ* **326**: 591–4

Solomon P (1992) Learning contracts in clinical education: evaluation by clinical supervisors. *Med Teach* **14**(2/3): 205–10

CHAPTER 3

Setting learning objectives

Judy McKimm and Tim Swanwick

Clinical teachers may be involved with students and trainees on a variety of different programmes who are required to achieve a diverse range of learning outcomes or objectives. Teachers who better understand the relationship between learning outcomes and the planning and delivery of educational activities can help learners receive more from their education and training.

This chapter explores the role of the clinical teacher in setting learning objectives for students or trainees in the context of the different curricula they may be following. It considers the roles of the individuals and organizations involved – the learner, the teacher and professional and healthcare organizations – alongside some core principles for writing clear and achievable learning objectives.

Aims, objectives and outcomes

Medical education uses a range of terms – aims, learning outcomes, learning objectives, competencies – to describe what learners should achieve as a result of educational interventions. This can be confusing, but it is often important that end points are clearly defined before the learning takes place. It is like planning a journey – if you don't know where you intend to go before you start, you may end up somewhere you don't want to be.

An aim usually defines what the programme or teacher is trying to achieve overall. It tells participants what the programme or session is about. For example: 'the aim of this session is to revise the principles of resuscitation and test your learning with a quiz'.

Learning objectives state the observable and measurable behaviours that learners should exhibit as a result of participating in a learning programme. An example of a learning (or instructional) objective would be: 'on completion of this course, the learner should be able to describe the common causes of a unilateral headache in an adult'.

Latterly, there has been a shift from defining such specific instructional objectives to providing more broad-based learning outcomes that are intended to arise as a result of the programme.

Harden (2002) suggests that learning outcomes are essentially more 'intuitive and user-friendly' than objectives: they are 'broad statements... that recognise the authentic interaction and integration in clinical practice of knowledge, skills and attitudes and the artificiality of separating these'. We can also view outcomes as learner goals. An example of this broader based approach might be:

'Graduates must know about biological variation, and have an understanding of scientific methods, including both the technical and ethical principles used when designing experiments'
(General Medical Council, 2003).

Increasingly, particularly at postgraduate level, learners are required to demonstrate specific competencies. An example around history taking at 1st year foundation trainee level might be that the doctor:

'routinely undertakes structured interviews ensuring that the patient's concerns, expectations and understanding are identified and addressed or demonstrates clear history taking and communication with patients' (The Foundation Programme, 2007).

In practice, the terms 'objectives', 'outcomes' and 'competencies' are often used interchangeably. Grant (2007) notes that it is fitness for purpose that is important and that the main purposes of stating intended learning achievements are to:

- Inform learners of what they should achieve
- Inform teachers about what they should help learners to achieve
- Form the basis of the assessment system, so that everyone knows what will be assessed
- Reflect accurately the nature of the profession into which the learner is being inducted and the professional characteristics that must be acquired.

Defining outcomes also helps us achieve what Biggs (1996) calls 'constructive alignment', where objectives, teaching methods and assessments are aimed at delivering the same thing. It is not just in face-to-face teaching that learning outcomes need to be aligned; learning materials, library and online support all have to be constructed to help the learner achieve the specified outcomes of the training programme.

Hierarchies of intended outcomes

In formal education, learning generally takes place within a predetermined framework where the specificity of outcomes at each stage increases towards the bottom of an educational hierarchy (*Figure 3.1*). For example, the General Medical Council defines very broad outcomes in the documentation

Figure 3.1. Levels at which learning outcomes may be defined.

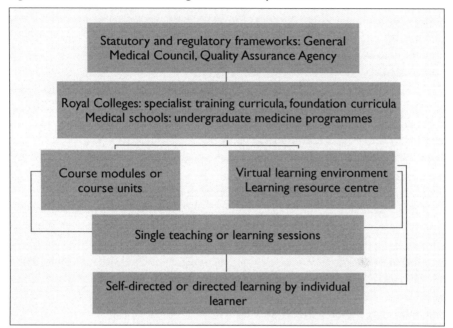

that supports the training of medical students. In the latest edition of *Tomorrow's Doctors* (GMC 2009) the GMC presents an outline curriculum under three broad headings, relating to the doctor as a scientist and scholar, a practitioner and a professional. Each category covers the development of the knowledge, skills and behaviour that the GMC wishes to see students demonstrate by the time they graduate.

Such overarching statements are interpreted and developed further by Royal Colleges and medical schools to generate curricula, often defined as broad outcomes, but which are then developed into much more specific objectives at programme, course, module and unit level, often framed in terms of knowledge, skills and professional attitudes. For foundation and specialty training programmes, learning outcomes may be defined in generic terms as well as more specifically related to the clinical context and level. At the level of the individual teaching episode, further specificity arises as the intended outcomes of a particular educational intervention, teaching or supervision session, are tailored to the needs of individual learners.

Prescription or process?

Learning outcomes or objectives can be seen as the building blocks of any learning programme or teaching or learning event and as key to ensuring that all aspects of a programme – learning methods, assessment, evaluation and quality assurance – link together. The teacher's role is to ensure that each session integrates with the whole curriculum by providing opportunities for learners to achieve the stated objectives and thus be capable of passing assessments.

When planning a session or programme, paying attention to how the outcomes will be achieved, assessed and evaluated requires active and overt consideration of the educational process: the interaction of teachers, students and knowledge. Stenhouse (1975) thought of an objective-led curriculum as an educational 'straitjacket', proposing a shift to a process-driven model in which the facilitation of learning is the central concern, and outcomes become unpredictable. Hussey and Smith (2008) call this the 'corridor of tolerance', allowing space for learning outcomes to emerge through the learning process. A thoughtful curriculum includes outcomes with varying levels of detail, enabling achievement of tasks, while acknowledging the importance of the process of learning. Medical curricula are now re-emphasizing the importance of students and trainees having opportunities to become immersed in clinical contexts, learning through experience. An example of a process objective might be: 'to spend time with the district nurse and explore how the service works.'

Learning objectives and professional development

Two models help us understand how learning outcomes or objectives relate to learners' professional development as they move from novice to expert.

Bloom

The first is found in Bloom's taxonomy of objectives in the cognitive domain (1956), which describes how objectives related to cognitive development increase in complexity as learners develop deeper understanding, start to apply this knowledge and ultimately synthesize and evaluate what they have learned. From your own experience you will know that as your clinical understanding developed, you became better able to handle complex information from multiple sources and synthesize it quickly and precisely to make consistently accurate diagnoses and decisions. Although this runs counter to experiential learning approaches in which learning happens by 'doing' (Kolb, 1984), Bloom's taxonomy has been highly influential in all areas of education.

Figure 3.2. Thinking like a professional? Bloom's taxonomy and professional development.

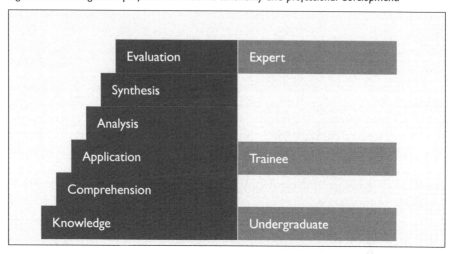

Figure 3.2 shows how these levels increase in complexity as learners advance. Bloom's model can be used to help write objectives or outcomes where they can be mapped on to the appropriate level, depending on what learners are expected to achieve. A common mistake in writing outcomes is to set them at the wrong level; either expecting learners to be able to do something for which they are not yet ready, or inappropriately linking them to particular teaching and learning methods or assessments.

Miller

Another model that is particularly useful for thinking about learning outcomes in relation to assessment of clinical competence is Miller's pyramid (1990) (*Figure 3.3*). This model is similar to Bloom's taxonomy in that there is a marked shift, as professionals develop expertise, from being able to demonstrate the knowledge underpinning competence (e.g. knowing theoretically how to examine an abdomen) to 'doing in action', where knowledge, skills and professional attitudes are synthesized and internalized into a seamless routine that can be carried out in different contexts.

Both these models can help us to match learning outcomes with our expectations of what the learner should be able to do at any stage. Students and trainees relate to knowledge and understanding at a more basic level – possibly in artificial or limited contexts – than to the actual high-level performance expected of consultants.

Figure 3.3. Miller's pyramid for assessing clinical competence. Adapted from Norcini (2007).

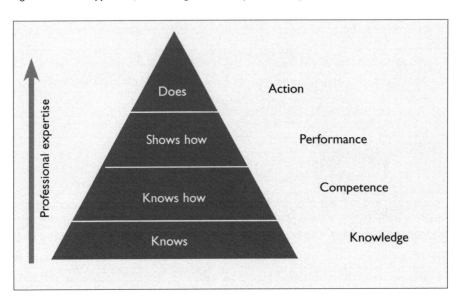

Writing learning outcomes or objectives

Learning objectives will relate to one of the three domains described by Bloom (1956):

1. Cognitive (knowledge and intellectual skills)
2. Psychomotor (physical skills)
3. Affective (feelings and attitudes).

They specify the intended end point of engagement in a given learning activity and:

- Are written in the future tense
- Use easily understood language
- Relate to explicit statements of achievement and always contain verbs
- Clearly indicate the nature and/or level of learning required for achievement
- Avoid ambiguity or over-complexity
- Are SMART: specific, measurable, achievable, realistic and timebound.

When writing objectives, always start with a stem, such as: 'At the end of this session, learners will be able to...' then use a verb, that states specifically what the learners will be able to do, e.g. '...demonstrate...' followed by a clear statement of the topic of interest '...that they can administer an intramuscular injection'.

Table 3.1 Writing objectives in the cognitive domain

	Description	Useful verbs for outcome level statements
Knowledge	Recall of information previously presented	Define, list, name, recall, record
Comprehension	Grasping the meaning but not extending it beyond the present situation	Describe, explain, discuss, recognize
Application	Using the rules and principles	Apply, use, demonstrate, illustrate, practice
Analysis	Breaking down components to clarify	Distinguish, analyse, calculate, test, inspect
Synthesis	Arranging and assembling elements into a whole	Design, organize, formulate, propose
Evaluation	Ability to judge X for a purpose	Judge, appraise, evaluate, compare, assess

Knowledge objectives

When writing objectives that relate to knowledge, there are a number of useful verbs that can be used to map the learning outcome onto the relevant tier of Bloom's taxonomy (*Table 3.1*). An example might be: 'At the end of this session, learners will be able to describe the key features of hypertension in adults'. For this learning objective, typical teaching and learning methods might be a lecture, seminar, tutorial, problem-based learning case or clinical scenario. We are not asking the learners to apply knowledge, therefore assessment would aim to assess understanding and recall of the key features of hypertension in adults.

Skills objectives

Bloom suggested that skills objectives should be written in terms of competence. He called this the psychomotor domain (although this taxonomy was completed by others) and ascribed to it five levels:

1. Imitation (observes skill and tries to reproduce it)
2. Manipulation (performs skill from instruction)
3. Precision (reproduces skill with accuracy and proportion)
4. Articulation (combines one or more skills in sequence with harmony and consistency)
5. Naturalization (completes skilful tasks competently and automatically).

Note the similarity to Miller's pyramid.

An example of a skills-based objective at the level of 'precision' would be: 'At the end of the training session, learners will be able to insert a cannula into a peripheral vein accurately without causing a haematoma'. Teaching and learning methods for this domain may well include some background knowledge, such as relevant anatomy and physiology or equipment needs, but for learners to be able to perform this skill accurately, they need to practise. This may be on models, or with supervision and feedback. Assessment of competence would involve a number of observations, not just asking the learner to describe what he/she would do.

Attitudinal objectives

Attitudinal objectives are often seen as the most difficult to write because they describe patterns of observable behaviour. Bloom called this the affective domain and again it has five levels:
1. Receiving (aware of external stimuli, e.g. listening)
2. Responding (complies with expectations in response to stimuli)
3. Valuing (displays behaviour consistent with a single belief without coercion)
4. Organizing (shows commitment to a set of values by behaviour)
5. Characterizing (behaviour consistent with a value system).

An example in this domain (at the level of responding) might be: 'At the end of the communications skills course, learners will be able to demonstrate awareness of cultural differences in working with simulated patients in three different clinical scenarios.'

This learning objective focuses on the learners being able to show that they understand and can respond to different (pre-defined in this case) cultural issues that patients may present. This objective states clearly that learners are not expected to demonstrate this awareness outside a simulated context, so not in the 'real world' of the ward.

Lesson planning

It is at the level of the individual teaching session that clinical teachers need to integrate the learning needs of their students or trainees with defined learning objectives. This can be achieved by asking four fundamental questions when planning teaching (adapted from Spencer, 2003):
1. Who am I teaching? (The number of learners and their level)
2. What am I teaching? (The topic or subject, the type of expected learning, e.g. knowledge, skills or attitudes)

3. How will I teach it? (Teaching and learning methods, length of time available, location of teaching session, access to patients and resources)
4. How will I know if the students understand? (Informal and formal assessments, questioning techniques, feedback from learners).

You might also want to ask:

- What do they know already?
- Where have they come from and what are they going on to next?
- What do the learners want as a result of the teaching and how can I find this out?
- How can I build in sufficient flexibility to cope with emerging needs?

For each teaching session it helps to formulate a 'lesson plan'. This may be very detailed or a simple broad brush outline, but before each session you should:

- Define your aims and learning outcomes or objectives
- Think about the structure of the session and timing of activities
- Decide on the best teaching and learning methods to achieve learning outcomes
- List content and key topics, research more if needed
- Refine your lesson plan
- Identify learning resources and support materials
- Finalize any linked assessment or evaluation.

Common pitfalls and how to avoid them

Careful planning helps teachers avoid some common pitfalls when setting learning outcomes for teaching and learning activities. *Table 3.2* lists some ways teachers might avoid these.

Conclusions

Setting learning objectives is a central activity for clinical teachers and the concept of pre-determined intended outcomes underpins all teaching, learning and assessment activities. Opportunities for setting learning objectives arise in formal planned educational activities as well as in more informal 'moment to moment' situations. Clinical teachers can optimize teaching and learning opportunities that arise in daily practice and support learners' professional development, through an in-depth understanding of the programme of study in which the learner is engaged, effective lesson planning and a continuous consideration of learners' needs.

Table 3.2. Common pitfalls and how to avoid them

Some pitfalls	...and how to avoid them
Trying to achieve too much in one session	Plan the session carefully, and allow time for discussion, activities and reflection.
Trying to cover too many learning outcomes	Stick to a small number of learning outcomes (fewer than five) and be as specific as you can in terms of exactly what you are expecting the learners to be able to do at the end of the session.
Learning outcomes not linked to the programme or to learner needs and prior experience	Make sure you know and understand the programme outcomes, the assessments the learners are working towards and the expectations of you by course organizers, particularly the outcomes and assessments that relate specifically to your session(s). Include informal and formal activities that help you understand and identify the needs of the learners.
Learning outcomes defined at the wrong level	Think carefully about exactly what you are expecting the learners to be able to do, think about their 'learning journey': their prior learning and the stage they have reached.
Learning outcomes in the wrong domain	Split objectives that cover more than one domain and design the teaching to enable learners to achieve all the outcomes. If you are assuming that learners have the underpinning knowledge or earlier practice to carry out a complex skill, check it out, or break the skill down into sub-objectives.
Learning outcomes not specific enough	Practice writing them and think about how you might assess the objective.
Learning outcomes not linked to teaching and learning methods	Select the teaching and learning methods that help learners achieve the outcome, e.g. if skills, need demonstration, practice (simulation or real), possibly broken down into steps, and feedback, not just reading about it or watching a video.
Learning outcomes not linked to assessment	Link the learning outcomes to an assessment, i.e. how will you and the learner know that he/she has achieved the outcome satisfactorily? Make sure the assessment assesses the right domain, e.g. skills are assessed by practical clinical assessments such as objective structured clinical examinations.
Learning outcomes not practical nor feasible	Often there are too many learning outcomes specified to cover in the time available or with the number or stage of learners. Check out equipment, rooms, other resources and facilities.

Table 3.2. Common pitfalls and how to avoid them (cont)	
Learning outcomes not linked to evaluation, little capacity to and change	If you are told what the outcomes are rather than setting them for yourself, be aware of the process by which you can feed back to course organizers review about how the session has worked. Think about making the links between learning outcomes, teaching and learning methods, assessment and evaluation transparent so you can refresh the curriculum. Do not assume that learning outcomes are set in stone.

KEY POINTS

- Setting learning objectives underpins effective clinical teaching, helping to determine teaching, learning and assessment methods.

- Understanding the curriculum, learners' needs and the educational context is essential when planning teaching sessions.

- Learning outcomes may be defined in terms of broad goals, instructional objectives or competencies.

- Learning outcomes should be defined in terms of what the learner should be able to do as a result of an educational intervention.

- Intended outcomes should be SMART: specific, measurable, achievable, realistic and timebound.

References

Biggs J (1996) Enhancing learning through constructive alignment. *Higher Education* **32**: 347–64

Bloom BS, ed. (1956) *Taxonomy of Educational Objectives*. David McKay Company Inc,New York

General Medical Council (2009) *Tomorrow's Doctors*. General Medical Council, London

Grant J (2007) *Principles of Curriculum Design*. Association for the Study of Medical Education, Edinburgh

Harden RM (2002) Learning outcomes and instructional objectives: is there a difference? *Med Teach* **24**: 151–5

Hussey T, Smith P (2008) Learning outcomes: a conceptual analysis. *Teaching in Higher Education* **13**(1): 107–15

Kolb DA (1984) *Experiential Learning: experience as the source of learning and development*. Prentice Hall, Englewood-Cliffs, NJ

Miller G, ed. (1990) T*eaching and Learning in Medical School.* Harvard University Press, Cambridge, MA

Norcini J (2007) *Workplace-based Assessment in Clinical Training.* Association for the Study of Medical Education, Edinburgh

Spencer J (2003) ABC of learning and teaching in medicine: learning and teaching in the clinical environment. *BMJ* **326**: 591–4

Stenhouse L (1975) *An Introduction to Curriculum Research and Development.* Heinemann, London

The Foundation Programme (2007) *Curriculum.* www.foundationprogramme.nhs.uk/pages/home/key-documents (accessed 16 June 2009)

CHAPTER 4

Curriculum and course design

Judy McKimm and Mark Barrow

Clinical teachers may be involved in planning and developing courses and teaching sessions for different groups of students or trainees. Understanding the principles of curriculum development and design can help teachers provide the most appropriate educational interventions for their learners.

This chapter introduces curriculum design and course development, highlighting some of the main approaches and recent trends in medical and healthcare education. Many of the principles described apply in a range of contexts and to both large and small-scale activities.

Introduction

A curriculum defines the learning that is expected to take place during a course or programme of study in terms of knowledge, skills and attitudes. It specifies teaching, learning and assessment methods and indicates the learning resources required to support effective delivery. One of the primary functions of a curriculum is to provide a framework or design which enables learning to take place. A syllabus is the part of a curriculum that describes the content of a programme.

The written and published curriculum (e.g. course documentation including the prospectus, course guides or lecturers' handouts) is the official or formal curriculum. The formal curriculum should match the functional (delivered) curriculum and is distinguished from the hidden, unofficial or counter curriculum. The hidden curriculum describes aspects of the educational environment and student learning (such as values and expectations that students acquire as a result of going through an educational process) which are not formally or explicitly stated but which relate to the culture and ethos of an organization.

The curricular cycle

In developing a new programme, or modifying an existing one, there are a number of stages which should be completed within the curricular cycle (*Figure 4.1*).

The broad context

Curriculum design needs to reflect the educational, healthcare and professional context and the level of the learners and expected outcomes. In addition, educational theories (e.g. adult learning, student-centred learning, flexible learning and self-directed learning) may influence the overall programme philosophy and approach.

Table 4.1 indicates how medical education has moved from a more teacher-centred, didactic approach to a more student-centred and community-based approach.

Medical and healthcare curricula are informed by reports and recommendations of statutory bodies, benchmarking and professional standards (e.g. *Tomorrow's Doctors;* General Medical Council, 2009), or a syllabus, learning outcomes or competency statements (e.g. those produced for postgraduate medical education). These provide templates for curriculum design and form the backdrop for audit, review and inspection.

Figure 4.1. The curriculum development and implementation cycle.

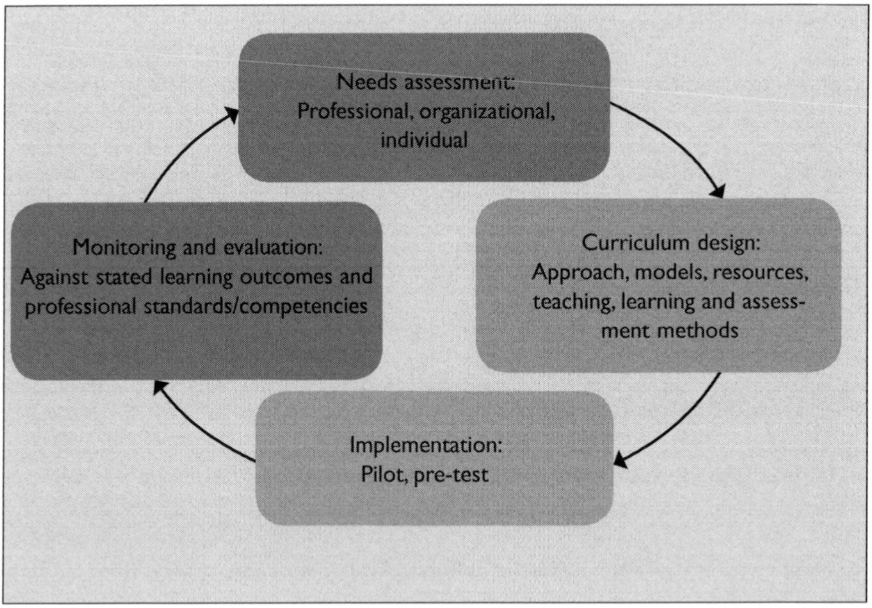

Curriculum strategies and approaches

All parts of a course or programme must fit (in terms of approach, level and content) with the overall course. When designing a new course, stakeholders' needs can be addressed through careful selection of educational approaches.

A strategic issue to consider is whether the course design, delivery and management is centrally managed or decentralized. Centralized curricula tend to be more structured and orderly and it is easier to ensure uniformity and a standard approach to teaching and learning. They may also allow better access to a wide pool of expertise but be less sensitive to local needs. Decentralized curricula can be more appropriate to students' local needs, enable a variety of approaches to design and delivery and ensure ownership of the course by teachers.

The objectives and the process models, which represent two philosophical approaches, have influenced curriculum development and design. They are not mutually exclusive.

Table 4.1 Trends in medical education	
Flexner (1910)	Teacher centred
	Knowledge giving
	Discipline led
	Hospital oriented
	Standard programme
	Opportunistic (apprenticeship)
Harden et al	Student-centred
(1984)	Problem-based
The SPICES model	Integrated
	Community oriented
	Electives (+ core)
	Systematic
Bligh et al (2001)	Practice based linked with professional development
PRISMS	Relevant to students and communities
	Interprofessional and interdisciplinary
	Shorter courses taught in smaller units
	Multisite locations
	Symbiotic (organic whole)

Objectives model

The objectives model defines learning in terms of what students should be able to do after studying the programme as learning outcomes or objectives.

Curriculum design according to this model follows four steps:

1. Reach agreement on broad aims and specific objectives for the course
2. Construct the course to achieve these objectives
3. Define the curriculum in practice by testing capacity to achieve objectives
4. Communicate the curriculum to teachers.

Objectives set at a superficial level or narrow specification limit the teacher and valuable learning experiences may be lost. Using an objectives model enables the construction of assessments which can be designed against the learning objectives. The objectives model reflects how national standards and curricula are described. It is a systematic approach to course planning and forms part of outcomes-based education (Prideaux, 2000) (*Figure 4.2*).

Process model

The process model sees content and learning activities as having intrinsic value, and not just as a means of achieving learning objectives. The model suggests that translating behavioural objectives is trivializing. Stenhouse (1975) suggests education comprises four fundamental processes:

1. Training (skills acquisition)
2. Instruction (information acquisition)
3. Initiation (socialization and familiarization with social norms and values)
4. Induction (thinking and problem solving).

He suggests that behavioural objectives are important only in the first two processes, that initiation and induction cannot be defined by using

Fig 4.2. The objectives or outcomes model.

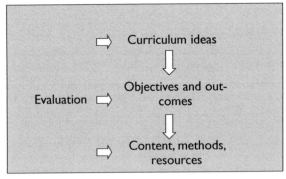

objectives and that behavioural objectives are inappropriate for problem-based learning, professional development or clinical problem solving.

The process model encourages creative or experiential approaches where learning is situated through experiences and group dynamics and outcomes emerge through the learning process (*Figure 4.3*).

Effective curriculum design combines both approaches according to student need, teacher experience and organizational structure and resources. For example, it is useful to design the overall shape of the course, the main aims and learning objectives, broad content areas and time allocation centrally but then devolve out the detailed planning and design to teachers who deliver the course so that they have ownership.

Models of curriculum design

In medical and healthcare education and training, learners are required to acquire a complex mix of knowledge, skills and attitudes, to be able to synthesize and apply their learning to new and often demanding situations and to be lifelong learners, acquiring and using skills and attitudes such as study skills and self motivation throughout their working lives.

Students need to acquire certain information or skills before they can move on to apply learning. The sequence of learning should move from simple 'building blocks' to understanding complex principles and enable the shift from 'novice' to 'expert'. The 'spiral curriculum' constructs learning as a developing process with active reinforcement and assessment at key stages coupled with the acquisition of new knowledge and skills. A learner-centred approach emphasizes adult learning methods, recognizing that learning is an active, constructive and contextually-bound activity. This takes the needs of individual and groups of learners into account, including factors such as gender, background, age and previous experience or education of the learners, learning styles or barriers to learning such as dyslexia or other disability. This approach

Figure 4.3. The process model.

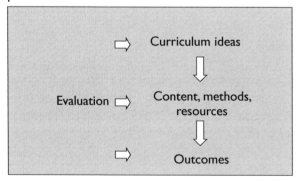

is more resource intensive as it relies on smaller groups, more advance planning is needed by teachers and students may need preparation in the shift from more didactic teaching.

To facilitate this, when planning or delivering a course or session, the teacher might ask:

- What level of understanding and experience do the learners have?
- What should I be expecting from the group in terms of knowledge, skills and attitudes?
- What topics and course areas have they been studying before this particular course or session?
- What are they going on to do and what should I be preparing them for?
- Have I built in opportunities for flexibility to address unforeseen learning needs?
- Where will the learning take place and what opportunities do the settings open up for me?
- Does the student or trainee have any particular learning needs or difficulties?
- How will I judge the effectiveness of my teaching as it progresses so that I can adjust the approach if necessary?

In undergraduate medical education, there are a few prevailing curricular models which embody different approaches to teaching and learning.

Pre-clinical and clinical model

The traditional pre-clinical and clinical model separates (both conceptually and temporally) pre-clinical knowledge and skills from clinical knowledge and skills. This was the prevailing model of medical education worldwide until the last 20 years and is still common across the world. Although the traditional approach has often been criticized for separating the underpinning 'science' from clinical medicine, it is often easier to develop and deliver a traditional course within the structure and organization of medical schools.

Graduate entry

Increasingly many medical courses are designed as graduate entry programmes, usually of about 4 years' duration, which build on students' earlier experiences and focus on clinical medicine. Students entering such courses would be expected to have obtained a good first degree in a relevant subject and passed an entry test.

Integrated curricula

Healthcare curricula are still subject centred but the overarching curriculum transcends traditional subject boundaries. Teaching units from subject disciplines are fused together around meaningful organizing themes or concepts. Vertical integration describes the blurring of boundaries between pre-clinical and clinical courses whereas horizontal integration describes how knowledge and skills from many disciplines are clustered around themes such as body systems (e.g. a cardiovascular systems course might include anatomy, physiology, biochemistry, pathology, clinical medicine, sociology and epidemiology). Integration helps students develop a more holistic view of patients' problems. However, some subjects or topics may be omitted or over taught and organizational boundaries such as departments and funding mechanisms may create barriers to integration. Close supervision and central curriculum mapping and management is required.

Problem-based learning

Problem-based learning has been very influential within medical education. Problem-based learning aims to stimulate students to observe, think, define, study, analyse, synthesize and evaluate a problem. The 'problems' or cases are written to simulate real-life clinical problems which are multidimensional and which encourage students to think as they would in real-life clinical situations. By addressing the 'problem' students learn to place propositional knowledge into 'real world' contexts, an approach that improves the retention and application of knowledge.

In practice a combination of models and methods is often most appropriate and most modern healthcare curricula synthesize different approaches.

Competencies

Clinical medicine at all levels tends to take a competency-based approach to the 'training' element of the curriculum although some critics note the reductionist approach to learning and assessment (e.g. Talbot, 2004). Competences are found in many areas of vocational training, where trainees are assessed against clearly stated competences (skills and procedures) to determine whether they are 'competent' or 'not yet competent'.

Decisions should be made on how 'threshold competence' will be determined and whether there are degrees of competence. For example, there would be widespread agreement that all medical graduates should be able to take blood or interpret an X-ray but there might be different expectations as to exactly what might be expected both from students at different stages of the course and as to the contexts and definitions of such competences. Assessments such as objective structured clinical examinations, mini clinical evaluation exercises or multisource feedback are widely used to gather evidence on which to make judgements about competence in clinical skills.

Key aspects of the curriculum

Any curriculum includes the following elements which must be 'constructively aligned' (Biggs, 1996):
- Aims
- Learning outcomes or objectives (knowledge, skills and attitudes)
- Content
- Teaching and learning methods
- Assessment methods.
- Supporting elements include:
- Learning resources (teachers, support staff, funding, books and journals, IT support, teaching rooms)
- Monitoring and evaluation procedures
- Clinical placement activities
- Recruitment and selection procedures, including promotional materials
- Student support and guidance mechanisms.

Aims and learning outcomes

Aims and learning outcomes or objectives need to ensure that the goal of producing competent graduates is achieved. Aims describe what the teacher is trying to achieve (e.g. to encourage students to develop self-directed learning skills) whereas goals usually describe what the course or organization is trying to achieve (e.g. to inculcate professional values and attitudes).

Learning outcomes guide teachers on what is expected of the learners on completion of the education or training programme, indicating the level at which a performance is expected. They also guide students on what they are expected to be able to do in terms of knowledge, skills and attitudes after completion (see Chapter 3).

One of the strengths of course planning using an objectives approach is that the objectives can be used as the measure for selecting teaching and learning methods and assessing student performance. Well-written objectives can be turned into assessment questions.

Curriculum content

Curriculum content comprises knowledge, skills, values and attitudes. Content should reflect the job that the learners will be asked to do after training, relate directly to learning outcomes, reflect balance between topics and theory and practice and be pitched at an appropriate level. Ideas for course content can be gathered from previous courses or existing curricula, national professional or discipline associations, textbooks, other organizations' courses on the internet and international bodies which have produced core curricula for their own subject.

Once the objectives or outcomes and broad content areas have been defined, the learning programme and timetable can be devised which allocates time for course elements and maps out a logical sequence of learning to enable student progression.

Teaching and learning methods

In many curricula, the choice of most appropriate teaching and learning methods is left up to the teacher. In others, such as problem-based learning curricula, the learning method is explicit in the curriculum design and guidelines will probably need to be produced to support teachers and students during the learning process.

Points to keep in mind are:
- How relevant are the teaching and learning methods to the content and learning outcomes?
- Where will the teaching and learning take place?
- How are practical skills going to be taught and supervised?
- How are students supported in independent learning and study (e.g. self-directed learning)?
- What resources are required and available to ensure effective teaching and learning?
- Does the teaching promote critical and logical thinking by the learner?
- What are the constraints affecting the teaching and learning process?
- Are the teaching and learning methods appropriate for the selected assessment methods?

Assessment methods

A curriculum sets out the assessment methods (as opposed to the actual assessment tasks) that will be used to measure students' performance. The starting point should always be the stated learning outcomes. Assessments must check that students have achieved the learning outcomes in various contexts and thus that the content has been covered. Teaching and learning methods must support the assessment strategy. An assessment blueprint (or matrix) maps out coverage of core content and learning outcomes against the assessment methods.

Teachers should check a number of aspects relating to assessment:

- Are the assessment methods which relate to the assessment of knowledge, skills and attitudes appropriate?
- Do the teaching and learning methods support the assessment strategy?
- Are the assessment methods reliable and valid?
- Are the assessment methods designed so that learners can achieve the minimum performance standards set in the curriculum and is there capacity for learners to demonstrate higher standards of performance (i.e. do the assessments enable discrimination between candidates)?
- Are there enough assessments or are learners being over-assessed?
- Are the regulations governing assessment procedures and awards clear and easy to follow and are they being applied appropriately and consistently?

Learning resources

The implementation of a new course usually requires additional learning resources or at least a rethink of existing learning resources. Teachers need to be aware of the resources available as part of course planning including staff, technical and administrative staff, equipment, budget and funding, books, journals and multimedia resources, teaching rooms, office space, social and study space and requirements for supervision and delivery of clinical teaching.

Implementing the curriculum

Once the curriculum has been fully developed it is ready for implementation. Those involved with implementation (usually teachers and examiners as well as students) need to interpret the curriculum in the same way as it is put into practice. Pre-testing or piloting can help to identify problems and issues and how a course works in practice. No course is perfect and one should always expect to continually modify and improve courses.

Monitoring and evaluation

Finally, the curriculum or course needs to be monitored and evaluated to ensure that it is working as planned and to identify areas for improvement. Evaluation involves ongoing formal feedback activities aimed at gathering timely information about the quality of a programme. It is important to build in evaluation activities to identify successes and failures of the curriculum with a view to correcting deficiencies, to measure if stated objectives have been achieved, to assess if the curriculum is meeting the needs of learners and the community and to measure the cost effectiveness of the curriculum. Monitoring and evaluation methods include observation, feedback questionnaires, focus groups, interviews, student assessment results and reports which the institution has to provide for internal use (e.g. absence statistics) or external agencies.

Conclusions

The act of preparing an effective course or curriculum provides an educator with a unique opportunity to consider, at the same time, the needs of patients, healthcare providers and professions, and learners and the interaction among them. A good curriculum recognizes that learning is an active, constructive and contextual process. It will provide guidance that helps educators to enable learners to acquire new knowledge and skills and apply them in a range of contexts.

The careful alignment of aims, learning outcomes, teaching approaches and assessment methods which is inherent in excellent curriculum design places educators in the best possible position to create an environment that supports student learning.

KEY POINTS

- A curriculum is an holistic statement that addresses the needs of all those involved in learning, from professions to teachers to students.
- It provides a template for planning and evaluating learning, teaching and assessment.
- Constructive alignment of aims, learning outcomes, teaching approaches and assessment methods supports good student learning.
- A cycle of needs assessment, curriculum design, delivery, review and evaluation results in a curriculum that keeps pace with the evolving needs of all stakeholders.
- Curriculum development principles can be applied at all levels of planning and design.

References

Biggs J (1996) Enhancing learning through constructive alignment. *Higher Education* **32***: 347–64*

Bligh J, Prideaux D, Parsell G (2001) PRISMS: new educational strategies for medical education. *Med Educ* **35:** 520–1

Flexner A (1910) *Medical Education in the United States and Canada: A Report to the Carnegie Foundation for the Advancement of Teaching*. Carnegie Foundation for the Advancement of Teaching, New York

General Medical Council (2009) *Tomorrow's Doctors 2009*. GMC, London

Harden RM, Sowden S, Dunn WR (1984) Educational strategies in curriculum development: the SPICES model. *Med Educ* **18:** 284–97

Prideaux D (2000) The emperor's new clothes: from objectives to outcomes. *Med Educ* **34:** 168–9

Stenhouse L (1975) *An Introduction to Curriculum Research and Development*. Heinemann, London: 52–83

Talbot M (2004) Monkey see, monkey do: a critique of the competency model in graduate medical education. *Med Educ* **38***: 1–7*

CHAPTER 5

Giving effective feedback

Judy McKimm

Feedback is a vital part of education and training which, if carried out well, helps motivate and develop learners' knowledge, skills and behaviours. It helps learners to maximize their potential and professional development at different stages of training, raise their awareness of strengths and areas for improvement, and identify actions to be taken to improve performance.

Introduction

This chapter sets out the principles behind giving effective feedback, considers different contexts in which feedback can be given and explores some of the issues involved in giving feedback to students, trainees and colleagues. It also provides suggestions on how you might apply these ideas to your own practice.

The role of feedback in clinical education

Many clinical situations involve the integration of knowledge, skills and behaviours in complex and often stressful environments with time and service pressures on both teacher and learner. Feedback is central to developing learners' competence and confidence at all stages of their medical careers, with the most effective feedback being that based on observable behaviours (Gordon, 2003).

Over the last few years, new assessment procedures have been introduced for doctors. Clinical practice and professional behaviours and attitudes are regularly and routinely assessed using a raft of workplace-based assessments, including multisource feedback, observations of clinical performance and case-based discussions. Feedback is a critical element of all these assessments. Incorporating feedback within learning that emphasizes reflective practice helps learners to develop the capacity to critically evaluate their own and others' performance, to self monitor and move towards professional autonomy.

Feedback and the learning process

Feedback can be informal, in day-to-day encounters between teachers and students or trainees, between peers or colleagues, or formal, for example as part of written or clinical assessment of learners' performance. Giving and asking for feedback should be part of the overall interaction between teacher and learner, not a one-way communication.

If feedback is not given, the learner might assume that he/she has no areas for improvement or development. Learners value feedback, especially when given by someone whom they respect for their knowledge, attitudes or clinical competence. Failing to give feedback is in itself a non-verbal communication, leading to mixed messages and false assessment by the learner of his/her own abilities as well as a lack of trust in the teacher or clinician. Feedback should also be aligned with the overall learning outcomes of the programme, teaching session or clinical activity in which the learner is engaged.

Kolb (1984) proposed that learning happens in a circular fashion, i.e. that learning is experiential (learning by doing) with ideas being formed and modified through experiences (*Figure 5.1*). The learning cycle moves through four phases:

1. Concrete experience – learners are enabled and encouraged to become involved in new experiences
2. Reflective observation – learners reflect on their learning
3. Abstract conceptualization – learners form and process ideas and integrate them with their existing cognitive frameworks
4. Active experimentation – learners use theories and frameworks to solve problems and test out in new situations.

Figure 5.1. Kolb's learning cycle. From Kolb (1984).

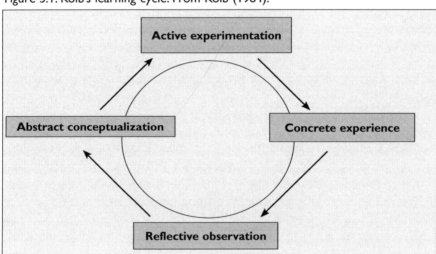

This cycle is similar to the 'plan, do, reflect, act' cycle which is often used in appraisals.

Hill (2007) identifies the important role of feedback in the learning cycle, in supporting reflection and considering how theory relates to practice. Clinical teachers can work with learners to negotiate and plan future learning needs and experiences. In order to help learners achieve their learning goals we need to start with an understanding of:

1. Where the learner is 'at', the level he/she has reached, his/her past experience and understanding of learning needs and goals
2. The learning goals in terms of know-ledge, technical skills and attitudes: you may be observing more than one of these learning domains at the same time (Hill, 2007).

During any observation, teachers need to be able to identify where and how far the learner has travelled towards the learning goals, where he/she may have gone off track and what further learning or practice may be required.

Giving effective feedback

Whether you are giving formal or informal feedback, applying some basic principles will help your feedback to be more effective.

Feedback should be given when asked to do so or when your offer is accepted and as soon after the event as possible. The overall focus is on the positive and should be part of the overall communication process and 'developmental dialogue'. To be effective it is important to develop rapport, mutual respect and trust between you and the learner.

Feedback needs to be given privately wherever possible, especially more negative feedback and in doing so, try to stay in the 'here and now'. Don't bring up old concerns or previous mistakes, unless this is to highlight a pattern of behaviours but focus on specific behaviours that can be changed, not personality traits, giving examples where possible and do not evaluate or assume motives. Use 'I' (i.e. own the feedback yourself) and give your experience of the behaviour (When you said..., I thought that you were...). When giving negative feedback, it is essential to suggest alternative behaviours.

Remember that feedback is for the recipient, not the giver: be sensitive to the impact of your message. Consider the content of the message, the process of giving feedback and the congruence between your verbal and non-verbal messages. Aim to encourage reflection through open questions such as:

- Did it go as planned – if not why not?
- If you were doing it again what would you do the same next time and what would you do differently... why?

- How did you feel during the session…how would you feel about doing it again?
- How do you think the patient felt…what makes you think that?
- What did you learn from this session?

When giving feedback to individuals or groups, an interactive approach helps to develop a dialogue between the learner and the person giving feedback. It builds on the learner's own self-assessment and helps learners take responsibility for learning. A structured approach ensures that both trainees and trainers know what is expected of them during the feedback sessions.

A number of different models have been developed for giving feedback in a structured and positive way. The simplest of these is a chronological statement of your observations, replaying the events that occurred during the session back to the learner. This can be helpful for short feedback sessions, but can become bogged down in detail during long sessions. Other models include the 'feedback sandwich' which starts and ends with positive feedback, with the aspects for improvement 'sandwiched' in between and 'Pendleton's rules' (Pendleton et al, 1984). Be clear about what you are giving feedback on and link this to the learner's overall professional development and/or intended programme outcomes. Finally, do not overload the learner – identify two or three key messages that you summarize at the end.

Barriers to giving effective feedback

Hesketh and Laidlaw (2002) identify a number of barriers to giving effective feedback in the context of medical education:

- A fear of upsetting the trainee or damaging the trainee–doctor relationship
- A fear of doing more harm than good
- The trainee being resistant or defensive when receiving criticism
- Feedback being too generalized and not related to specific facts or observations
- Feedback not giving guidance as to how to rectify behaviour
- Inconsistent feedback from multiple sources
- A lack of respect for the source of feedback.

Increasingly in medical education, a range of health professionals and patients are involved in formal assessments, either in the workplace or in more formal settings. This can cause anxieties and barriers for both those giving and receiving feedback. Feedback needs to be sensitively and appropriately given. It is easy for those giving feedback to:

*'take the relationship aspect of their roles for granted... particularly if the
(teacher) has been working with their learner for some time'
(Parsloe, 1995).*

Learners are often in a dependent and subordinate role to teachers or trainers
and it is easy to dismiss issues of organizational power and authority that
often underpin work relationships. This is particularly important where there
may be tensions around professional role boundaries and status.

The person giving feedback and the recipient might be different in terms
of sex, age or educational and cultural background. Although these might
not pose obstacles they may make some feedback sessions strained and
demotivating. A supportive, empathic, consistent and relaxed environment
and a working relationship based on mutual respect is the basis for enabling
feedback to be most effective and helps the learner take responsibility for
development and improvement.

Informal feedback

Opportunities for giving informal feedback to learners can be taken through
questioning techniques, planning appropriate learning activities and building
in time for discussion (Spencer, 2003). *Table 5.1* indicates how feedback on
performance or understanding can be built into everyday practice, helping
learners move through the 'novice to expert' stages in the 'competency
model' of supervision (Proctor, 2001; Hill, 2007).

Providing informal 'on the job' feedback might take only a few minutes
of your time but to be most effective, the feedback should take place at the
time of the activity or as soon as possible after so that those involved can
remember events accurately. The feedback should be positive and specific,
focussing on the trainee's strengths and helping to reinforce desirable
behaviour: 'You maintained eye contact with Mrs X during the consultation,
I feel this helped to reassure her...'. Clinicians are influential role models.
Modelling how reflective practitioners behave by 'unpacking' your own
clinical reasoning and decision-making processes as you give feedback can
be an effective approach to developing a professional conversation.

Negative feedback should also be specific and non-judgmental, possibly
offering a suggestion: 'Have you thought of approaching the patient in
such a way...'. Focus on some of the positive aspects before the areas for
improvement: 'You picked up most of the key points in the history, including
X and Y, but you did not ask about Z...'. Avoid giving negative feedback in
front of other people, especially patients.

Keep the dialogue moving with open-ended questions: 'How do you
think that went?', which can be followed up with more probing questions.

Table 5.1 The role of feedback in professional development

	Unconscious incompetence	Conscious incompetence	Conscious competence	Unconscious competence
Learner	Low level of competence. Unaware of failings	Low level of competence. Aware of failings but not having full skills to correct them	Demonstrates competence but skills not fully internalized or integrated. Has to think about activities, may be slow	Carries out tasks without conscious thought. Skills internalized and routine. Little or no conscious awareness of detailed processes involved in activities
Role of feedback	Helps learner to recognize weaknesses, identify areas for development and become conscious of incompetence	Helps learner to develop and refine skills, reinforces good practice and competence, demonstrates skills	Helps learner to develop and refine skills, reinforces good practice and competence through positive regular feedback	Raise awareness of detail and unpack processes for more advanced learning, note any areas of weakness or bad habits

You should encourage learners to be proactive in seeking feedback from others as this is often more timely and relevant to learners' needs (Hesketh and Laidlaw, 2002).

Giving formal feedback

Clinicians are often required to give formal feedback based on observations of learners over a period of time, for specific purposes (e.g. appraisal, end of attachment interviews) or as part of assessment or revalidation. If ongoing feedback has been regularly carried out then formal feedback should not contain any surprises for the learners. Feedback can be given on a one-to-one basis or in small groups. The structure for giving feedback will be agreed between you and the learner(s). It is important that both you and those to whom you are giving feedback are fully prepared.

Before a formal feedback session you should:
- Ensure the learner is aware he/she is to receive feedback (so clearly define the purpose of the feedback session before or at the outset of the session)
- Collect any information you need from other people
- Summarize the feedback and ensure you know the positive aspects and areas for improvement are listed (with supporting evidence)
- Make sure you know how the feedback relates to the learning programme and defined outcomes.

Then set the scene:
- Create an appropriate environment
- Clarify ground rules, e.g. what part of the history or examination the learner is to concentrate upon, when you will interrupt, what other learners might do, how the learner can seek help during the consultation
- Agree a teaching focus
- Gain the patient's consent and cooperation
- Make notes of specific points.

During the formal feedback session, you should:
- Redefine the purpose and duration of the feedback session
- Clarify the structure of the session
- Encourage the learner to self assess his/her performance before giving feedback
- Aim to encourage dialogue and rapport
- Reinforce good practice with specific examples
- Identify, analyse and explore potential solutions for poor performance or deficits in practice.

After the session, you should:
- Complete any outstanding documentation and ensure you both have copies
- Carry out any agreed follow-up activities or actions
- Make sure that opportunities for remedial work or additional learning are arranged
- Set a date for the next feedback session if required (*Table 5.2*).

Receiving feedback

Sometimes feedback is not received positively by learners and fear of this can inhibit teachers giving regular face-to-face feedback. People's responses to criticism varies, however constructively it is framed. Learners often discount their ability to take responsibility for their learning and their responses may present in negative ways, including anger, denial, blaming or rationalization (King, 1999). It is useful to think in a structured way about how feedback might be received and to encourage an open dialogue and receptivity.

Table 5.2 Do's and don't's of effective feedback

Do:	Find an appropriate time and place
	Agree what you are going to focus on
	Start with what went well – accentuate the positive
	Distinguish between the intention and the effect
	Distinguish between the performance and the personal (e.g. 'what you said sounded judgmental' rather than 'you are judgmental'
	Identify areas for improvement
	Offer alternatives
	Check for understanding
Don't:	Generalize
	Comment on things that can't be changed
	Criticize without making recommendations
	Be dishonestly kind – if there is room for improvement be specific
	Forget that your feedback says as much about you as about the person to whom it is directed

Conclusions

Being able to give effective feedback on performance in both formal and informal settings is one of the key skills of a clinical teacher. Giving feedback can range from simple, informal questions and responses while working alongside a learner on a day-to-day basis through to giving written or verbal feedback through appraisal or examinations. However, the core principles are the same: a good relationship and dialogue helps the learner receive messages appropriately and the feedback should be given so as to help the learner take informed action and responsibility for their future learning and development.

KEY POINTS

- The skill of giving feedback is central to effective clinical teaching and supervision.
- The process of feedback is closely linked to learning and professional development.
- Feedback should always be constructive – focussing on behaviours that can be changed.
- Informal feedback can easily be built into everyday clinical practice.
- Developing a good relationship with learners helps feedback to be received more appropriately.

References

Gordon J (2003) BMJ ABC of Learning and Teaching in Medicine: One to one teaching and feedback. *BMJ* **326**: 543–5

Hesketh EA, Laidlaw JM (2002) Developing the teaching instinct: Feedback. *Med Teach* **24**(3): 245–8

Hill F (2007) Feedback to enhance student learning: Facilitating interactive feedback on clinical skills. *International Journal of Clinical Skills* **1**(1): 21–4

King J (1999) Giving feedback. *BMJ* **318**: 2

Kolb DA (1984) *Experiential Learning: Experience as the Source of Learning and Development*. Prentice Hall, Englewood-Cliffs, NJ

Parsloe E (1995) *Coaching, Mentoring and Assessing: A Practical Guide to Developing Competence*. Nichols Publishing, London

Pendleton D, Schofield T, Tate P, Havelock P (1984) *The Consultation: an Approach to Learning and Teaching*. Oxford University Press, Oxford

Proctor B (2001) Training for supervision attitude, skills and intention. In: Cutcliffe J, Butterworth T, Proctor B, eds. *Fundamental Themes in Clinical Supervision*. Routledge, London

Spencer J (2003) BMJ ABC of Learning and Teaching in Medicine: Learning and teaching in the clinical environment. *BMJ* **326**: 591–4

CHAPTER 6

Supervision

Helen Halpern and Judy McKimm

This chapter discusses the principles of supervision and the role of educational and clinical supervisors in supporting students, trainees and colleagues in a range of contexts. It also suggests how you might apply these principles to your own practice as a clinical teacher, and how you might further develop your supervision skills.

What is supervision?

If 'vision' implies seeing, the word 'supervision' can be read as over-seeing, looking over someone's shoulder to check on them, and also 'super' in the sense of outstanding or special: helping someone to extend their professional skills and understanding. Supervision supports professional learning and development, but also relates to monitoring and improving performance as part of effective clinical governance and standard setting.

In medical education, a distinction is often made between the two closely related activities of clinical and educational supervision (*Figure 6.1*).

Figure 6.1. Domains of supervision. From Launer (2006a).

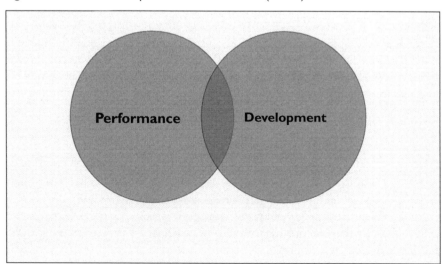

Educational supervision

Educational supervision is 'the provision of guidance and feedback on matters of personal, professional and educational development in the context of a trainee's experience of providing safe and appropriate patient care' (Kilminster et al, 2007). All doctors are required to have educational supervision across their whole training period (Department of Health, 2007) aimed at helping learners to develop self-sufficiency in acquiring skills and knowledge through meetings, observation of practice, assessments and the provision of pastoral care. It is important that the educational supervisor flags up any concerns at an early stage.

Clinical supervision

Clinical supervision relates to the everyday supervision of a trainee's performance. It involves being available, looking over the shoulder of the trainee and teaching on-the-job with developmental conversations, regular feedback and the provision of a rapid response to issues as they arise (Department of Health, 2007). All trainees must have a named clinical supervisor for each post who should tailor the level of supervision to the competence, confidence and experience of the trainee.

Clinical supervision is a core aspect of personal and professional development and lifelong learning, helping practising professionals develop complex skills in the context of real practical issues and situations which may include a variety of one-to-one professional encounters such as mentoring and coaching (Butterworth et al, 1996; Burton and Launer, 2003; Clark et al, 2006).

In the day-to-day clinical context, educational supervision necessarily includes some aspects of clinical supervision because issues discussed by the educational supervisor and supervisee often include aspects relating to clinical practice. Although educational supervision may cover some technical aspects of work, clinical supervision is the place where a wider range of issues around specific patients or dilemmas tends to be raised and addressed.

Mentoring, coaching and appraisal

Mentoring, coaching and appraisal are specific examples of supervision and involve a similar range of interpersonal and conversational skills:
- Mentoring is guidance and support provided by a more experienced colleague or through co-mentoring where colleagues meet to offer mutual support

- Coaching is a form of supervision aimed at unlocking someone's potential to maximize his/her performance (Launer 2006a)
- Appraisal is a formal process aimed at developing a person's professional performance, potential and ideas about career development (Peyton, 2000).

Benefits of supervision

Effective supervision uses the same skills as those applied in consultations with patients: respect, thoughtfulness, complexity, empowerment, use of open questions and being non-judgmental. Nursing studies indicate that good clinical supervision improves morale and job satisfaction and may prevent stress and burnout (Butterworth et al, 1996; Begat et al, 1997; Cutcliffe et al, 2001). In many emotionally demanding professions (such as psychotherapy and social work) practitioners at all stages of their careers are required to have ongoing professional supervision. Supervision also helps to promote reflective practice and contributes to professional development. In health care, professionals are increasingly required to demonstrate evidence of reflective practice as part of professional revalidation.

It is an example of the inverse care law (Hart, 1971) that those practitioners who are the most isolated and deprived are the least likely to receive any supervision. In other words, doctors who are least able to reflect on their work, either because they work alone, or because their psychological skills are less well developed, are the very practitioners who may most benefit from the opportunity to have supervision.

Preparing the ground

There are a number of underpinning principles for good supervisory practice:
1. Be clear about why there is a need for supervision and who has asked for it
2. Set a time frame for the supervision session – even a few minutes of focussed time can be worthwhile
3. Protect the time and space and ensure that professional confidentiality is maintained
4. Arrange seating to facilitate a conversation between peers
5. Clarify the extent to which the supervision is about development or performance.

Cases, contexts and careers

Most supervision conversations address the three inter-related domains of cases, contexts and careers. The role of the supervisor is clearer in some of these domains than others.

Cases

Clinical supervision can be particularly helpful in cases which involve:
- Ethical issues such as when it is unclear how to proceed with or stop investigations or treatment
- Complex decision-making because of the interaction of clinical, social and psychological factors
- Dealing with angry, distressed, unlikeable patients or their families
- Handling complaints or significant events
- Patients presenting with somatization, conditions where there is no clear diagnosis or patients who attend frequently.

Educational supervisors also need to be able to discuss clinical cases and know to whom the learner can be referred to discuss clinical issues that may require more expert knowledge. Discussing clinical cases may highlight patterns of behaviours through which educational needs are revealed which can be included in the learning contract. You might also advise on areas suitable for assessment or further practice or experience.

Contexts

Clinical scenarios depend on the place in which they occur, the players involved and the interactions between these people. Issues relating to contexts might include:
- Professional or interprofessional difficulties
- Communication problems
- Difficulties in teamwork
- Conflicts about roles or boundaries
- Differing expectations about care
- Power, authority, money or politics.

Educational supervisors need to understand the supervisee's work contexts as they relate to his/her learning needs, educational objectives and professional development. With the agreement of your supervisee, you may be required to mediate or discuss issues with others.

Careers

Supervision conversations can often raise issues about careers, including further training needs, work conditions, job prospects and career aspirations (including retirement), and how to manage and delegate work.

Educational supervision is key to this process and your role is to support learners on their 'learning journey' which, although having elements in common with that of other students or trainees, is unique to that person. Understanding the strengths, areas for development and aspirations of your supervisees will facilitate effective and timely supervision.

Constraints and challenges

Some supervision roles, such as educational supervision of trainees, have clearly defined outcomes and activities within established clinical and educational structures. Here you need to familiarize yourself with the obligations of the role and support available. The 'supervision' role may be looser in other contexts, such as where clinicians are responsible for medical students, healthcare students or professional colleagues. Here, you need to clarify expectations from learners and the organizations responsible for them as these may differ between organizations and with the level of the supervisee.

Other challenges include personal differences between supervisors and supervisees, based on age, gender, culture, sexuality, work or career patterns, seniority, qualifications, disability, speech, accent or domestic commitments. Sometimes differences can be used positively to help each challenge thinking and assumptions and promote creativity; at other times differences may lead to an unhelpful power imbalance which may constrain the supervision relationship. Active consideration of such issues can help you decide whether these should be discussed with your supervisee.

Power can impact on the supervisee to make him/her behave defensively and paralyse his/her ability to think; out of fear or excessive respect, supervisees may then simply accept your ideas without question. Sometimes you may feel particularly challenged, frustrated or de-skilled by certain supervisees. Although this does not happen frequently, if either of you feel that there is a 'clash' and that the supervision process is not working successfully, it is important to know where to seek help and advice. Ultimately, each of you may have a more helpful working relationship with a different person.

More general constraints to effective supervision include:
- Lack of time
- Worries about the possible enormity of the problem – opening a 'can of worms'
- Need for appropriate training to carry out supervision
- Embedded cultural attitudes: for some clinicians there is a tradition of working alone, taking individual responsibility, or training and supervision being given a low priority
- Fear of showing areas of weakness or need
- Anxiety about professional revalidation
- Attitudes about 'policing' the profession.

A narrative-based approach to supervision: the seven Cs

One aim of supervision is to help people to find new versions of a situation which has become stuck by asking questions which invite change. Palazzoli Selvini et al (1980) suggest that supervisors should not give advice, offer solutions or make interpretations. Educational supervision may, however, require a more directive approach such as asking questions which help people think from new angles (Tomm, 1988). These techniques, and ways of asking questions, have been formulated into core concepts (the 'seven Cs', adapted from Launer, 2006b), which illustrate how to put supervision into practice.

Conversations

Here the conversation itself is seen as the working tool. Effective conversations do not simply describe people's view of reality, they create new understanding of it through the opportunity for people to rethink and reconstruct their stories.

Curiosity

Curiosity changes chat into a more substantial conversation in which the story about patients, colleagues and oneself is developed. Supervisors need to pay close attention to verbal and non-verbal language used, and their own responses and feelings (such as criticism, boredom or anxiety). It is important to consciously take a neutral and non-judgmental stance which allows us become curious about different positions others might take, including the position of no change.

Contexts

This includes the person's networks, his/her sense of culture, faith, beliefs, community, values, history and geography and how these may impinge on the conversation. An important context is that of how power is understood. Who holds the power and how is this seen by others? Who is asking for supervision and for what purpose? The context helps the conversation come alive.

Complexity

This involves thinking about things in a non-linear way, getting away from fixed ideas of cause and effect, thinking about the interactions between people and the kind of patterns which develop between people and events over time to produce a richer description of the story.

Creativity

Creativity means finding a way to create a story or account of reality which makes better sense for people than the one they are going through. To do this involves using oneself, intuition and sensitivity to fine-tune the conversation. It also implies the creative process of jointly constructing a new version of the story.

Caution

This consists of looking for cues from the_supervisee to monitor his/her responses. It involves working on the cusp between affirmation and perturbation in order to challenge appropriately without being confrontational or too bland. Sometimes it is appropriate to give straightforward advice (although you need to be aware of its limitations).

Care

Being respectful, considerate and attentive to patients, your supervisee and yourself is important, as is ensuring that supervision and clinical activities are carried out ethically.

The supervision process

The process of supervision gives an opportunity for supervisees to reconstruct their view of a particular situation or issue through the supervisor asking questions to try to help them see things from different perspectives. This is part of an iterative process (*Figure 6.2*) which might take place within one session or over a period of time.

In order to help people come to their own conclusions and solutions it is often better to withhold advice until towards the end of the conversation. This does not mean that you should not tell a supervisee what to do, especially within an urgent clinical setting.

Some useful general questions to ask in supervision

- What would you like to happen or what do you want?
- How will you know if this piece of supervision has been helpful to you?
- What do I need to know about…?
- What do you see as the main issues or your chief dilemma?
- What do you think are the main contexts influencing this situation?
- How do you understand…?

Figure 6.2. The circular process of supervision.

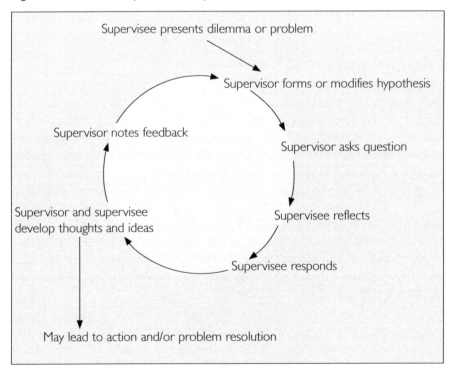

- What explanations do you have?
- How would you describe...?
- How would x view you or what is going on?
- What would x say?
- Has there been a situation like this before?
- When x does this what does y do or how would y react?
- What you have said made me curious about...
- How would a primary care trust manager, the General Medical Council or a lawyer regard this?
- If you looked at this from a 'patient safety' perspective what thoughts would you have?
- What are the differences in beliefs, understandings or approaches between...?
- What do you think would need to happen?
- What would happen if you tried...?
- Where do you think things will be in ... (time)?
- What will happen if nothing changes?

Conclusions

Supervision is essential in promoting professional development and ensuring effective clinical performance. These 'professional conversations' may take place informally over a snatched coffee break or popping in to a colleague's room, or formally in designated teaching sessions, tutorials or team meetings. Supervision is based on the core principles of mutual respect, a good working relationship and developing an open and honest conversation centred around the supervisee's educational and professional needs.

References

KEY POINTS

- Be clear about the context of supervision, the supervisor's role and the supervisee's needs in terms of development and performance.
- Think about what can realistically be achieved in the time available.
- Be aware of issues of professional confidentiality, clinical governance, power differences and ethics.
- Know who to go to in order to get personal supervision.
- Supervision is a part of lifelong learning and does not stop at the end of training.
- Good supervision contributes to job satisfaction, reflective practice and stress reduction, and improves patient care.

Begat I, Severinsson E, Berggren I (1997) Implementation of clinical supervision in a medical department: Nurses' views of the effects. *J Clin Nurs* **6**: 389–94

Burton J, Launer J, eds (2003) *Supervision and Support in Primary Care*. Radcliffe Medical Press, Oxford

Butterworth T, Bishop V, Carson J (1996) First steps towards evaluating clinical supervision in nursing and health visiting. 1. Theory, policy and practice development: a review. *J Clin Nurs* **5**: 127–32

Clark P, Jamieson A, Launer J, Trompetas A, Whiteman J, Williamson D (2006) Intending to be a supervisor, mentor or coach: which, what for and why? *Education for Primary Care* **17**: 109–16

Cutcliffe J, Butterworth T, Proctor B (2001) *Fundamental Themes in Clinical Supervision*. Routledge, London and New York

Department of Health (2007) *A guide to Postgraduate Speciality Training in the UK. The Gold Guide*. HMSO, London

Hart JT (1971) The Inverse care law. *Lancet* **i**: 405–12

Kilminster S, Cottrell D, Grant J, Jolly B (2007) AMEE Guide No.27: Effective educational and clinical supervision. *Med Teach* **29**: 2–19

Launer J (2006a) *Supervision, mentoring and coaching: one-to-one learning encounter in medical education*. Association for the Study of Medical Education, Edinburgh

Launer J (2006b) New stories for old: Narrative-based primary care in Great Britain. *Families, Systems and Health* **24**: 336–44

Palazzoli Selvini M, Boscolo L, Cecchin G, Prata G (1980) Hypothesizing, circularity, neutrality: Three guidelines for the conductor of the session, *Family Process* **19**(1): 3–12

Peyton JWR (2000) *Appraisal and Assessment in Medical Practice: A Practical Guide for Management and Staff*. Manticore Europe Ltd, Rickmansworth

Tomm K (1988) Interventive interviewing: Part III. Intending to ask lineal, circular, strategic or reflexive questions? *Family Process* **27**(1): 1–15

CHAPTER 7

Facilitating learning in the workplace

Clare Morris

Workplace-based learning has been at the heart of medical education and training for centuries. However, radical reform of the NHS means we have to re-think traditional approaches to apprenticeship and find new ways to ensure that students and trainees can learn 'on-the-job' while doing the job.

This chapter explores contemporary perspectives on workplace-based learning and considers how they guide learning in medical workplaces. Ways to create an environment where learning happens in parallel with working, are explored. In addition, strategies to maximize workplace-based learning are identified.

Learning in the workplace: Opportunities and challenges

The workplace offers rich opportunities for learning, enabling learners to develop professional knowledge, skills, behaviours and attitudes and work collaboratively to deliver patient care. Critically, it is the site of professional socialization, where professional identity is shaped. Finding ways to support such development while meeting patient needs is a challenge for clinical teachers. One way to address this is to put aside the types of teaching developed for the classroom and provide learning opportunities that are compatible with the workplace.

Clinical teachers identify the following challenges to workplace-based learning:

- Available time and resources
- Competing demands and priories
- Increased paperwork for training and assessment
- Changing expectations
- Concerns about the risks involved in delegating clinical work.

Students and trainees report concerns about lacking a clear role, knowing what is expected of them, limited opportunities to be observed and receive feedback on performance and, increasingly, being unclear about the inherent learning value of daily work activity.

Learning as participation

It is helpful to distinguish conceptions of learning as 'acquisition' (of knowledge or skills) from those that see learning as 'participation' in workplace practices and cultures (Bleakley, 2002; Swanwick, 2005). Learning as acquisition drives learners from the workplace into classrooms and leads to clinics and theatre lists over-running as clinicians attempt to 'teach' students between patients or procedures. Learning as participation opens up new opportunities for learning while working. In the 1980s, Kolb represented this type of learning as a cycle (see *Figure 5.1 on page 42*) which focussed on the types of experiences learners had and how they made sense of these experiences (Kolb, 1984). The influence of this type of thinking can be seen in the increasing use of case-based discussion as an assessment tool and in the wholesale adoption of 'reflective portfolios' in training.

Kolb's cycle provides a framework to consider what needs to happen beyond 'doing something' for learning to take place. This model poses two risks: implying that experiential learning is an individual pursuit divorced from context and downplaying the complexity of learning in and through experience and the role played by the clinical teacher.

Sociocultural learning theories

More recently, attention has turned to sociocultural theories of learning and concepts such as 'communities of practice' and 'situated learning' (Wenger, 1998; Lave and Wenger, 2003). These theories see learning not as an individual pursuit but as something that happens through engagement in shared activities and practices.

Drawing on this viewpoint, distinctions between medical learning and working are artificial creating implications for those who support learning in the workplace (Bleakley, 2002, 2006; Swanwick, 2005). So, for example, when clinicians gather round the bedside to talk to patients and discuss their progress and management with members of the team, they are engaged in both a working and learning activity. Their understandings of one another, their patients and their illnesses are influenced by the conversations around the bed and by the notes made, which become part of workplace-based learning.

Clinical teachers therefore need to make this learning more explicit to trainees, to help them recognize that they are learning 'how to do the job' by 'doing the job'. The extent to which it is possible to learn through work activity is influenced by recognizing and making explicit the learning embedded in everyday practice.

Facilitating learning in the workplace

In the following sections, key ideas arising from these theories are identified and the implications for practice explored.

Learning is part of everyday life

If learning is seen as an integral part of working, clinical teachers need to make the learning more explicit by identifying specific workplace cultures and practices and helping learners 'make sense' of what they see, hear, sense and do. Strategies include:

- Label the learning opportunity, e.g. 'we have a theatre list this afternoon and we need to consent patients this morning. It would be a great opportunity for you to learn more about how to explain procedures and gaining patient consent.'
- Establish prior experience and negotiate a learning goal, e.g. 'so, you have experience of consenting patients for routine procedures, so why don't we work together this morning to consent patients about to undergo more complex procedures, with the aim being that you will be able to do this independently next time?'
- Prime for learning through observing, e.g. 'in clinic this morning we are likely to see patients who are booked in for caesarean section. While you observe, notice the reasons given for requesting elective section and consider how you would respond if in my shoes.'
- Workplace-based assessment tools can be used to identify opportunities for learning and development through workplace-based activity, e.g. 'I noticed you were struggling with putting in that line, why don't you arrange to work with one of the anaesthetists for the day and get some extra experience in theatre?'

Workplaces need to be made 'invitational'

Students and trainees who are made to feel welcome are more likely to actively engage in the full range of learning opportunities provided and to seek to play an active role in the team. Simple strategies like ensuring students are introduced by name, have a period of orientation to the workplace and the roles of other team members can make a big difference. Billett (2002, 2004) suggests that workplaces are not necessarily 'invitational' to all learners, and may be shaped, for example, by students' prior experiences, their gender, socioeconomic background or apparent differences in motivation, enthusiasm or interest.

Clinical teachers need to create the right conditions for learning and ensure certain types of learners are not disadvantaged. For example, trainees who seem to lack interest, confidence or capability for a particular specialty need just as much opportunity to participate (if not more) than those who have a natural flair or interest.

Learning in a community of practice

Teams can be seen as potential 'communities of practice' (Lave and Wenger, 2003), identified by common interests and shared expertise. To make the most of that expertise, all members of the community should be engaged in supporting learning. Learners readily identify colleagues, team members, patients and carers who help them 'fit in' to new settings and who make positive contributions to their learning. These individuals may not have a formally recognized teaching role, for example:

- Patient feedback is very powerful in reinforcing practice or seeking new ways to do things
- Students and trainees learn from each other (e.g.'I find it helpful to hold it this way') and share experiences (e.g.'I saw a great case in theatre yesterday')
- Junior medical staff guide less experienced colleagues in ways of examining patients, interpreting charts or test results and prioritizing workloads
- Nursing colleagues help newcomers get to grips with ward procedures and protocols and identify ways to effectively work with particular team members.

By acknowledging the role played by all members of your community and valuing it explicitly, learners are encouraged to look beyond their immediate supervisor for guidance.

Learning happens through participation

Learning is most effective when learners are given opportunities to engage actively in real workplace activity. Such opportunities are bounded by competing demands, concerns and priorities, the complexity of the activity, the potential risks involved, the competence and confidence of the learner, the time available and the willingness (and consent) of patients to be involved. With adequate preparation and 'safety netting', clinical teachers can delegate some complete tasks to learners whereas other opportunities require teachers to work in parallel with learners, delegating appropriate aspects of work in order to increase confidence and competence.

One of the ways in which teachers can 'safety net' is through learning needs analysis (see Chapter 2). A brief yet really focussed conversation with a trainee can inform decision making about what to delegate and appropriate support strategies. This will usually include finding out what the trainee knows, what he/she has done before that is of relevance, any concerns or anxieties he/she has about what is proposed and an offer of back-up support (a rescue strategy) to be used if things don't go according to plan.

For example, a trainee might not yet be ready to perform a complete surgical procedure. He/she may, however, be ready to take the history, perform the examination, consent the patient, prep the patient and perform one part of the procedure, monitor in recovery and write up the charts. This gives the trainee a sense of taking responsibility for the patient's management and time to focus his/her attention fully on the aspects he/she is not yet doing, but might do next time.

Workplace-based assessments provide a profile of trainee performance, enabling the clinical teacher to spot obvious gaps in either experience or competence. These gaps can become the focus on clinical teaching, with the trainee being guided to experiences that help meet their development needs.

Fostering 'horizontal' learning

'Learning in work-based contexts involves students having to come to terms with a dual agenda. They not only have to learn how to draw upon their formal learning and use it to interrogate workplace practices; they also have to learn how to participate in workplace activities and cultures' *(Griffiths and Guile, 1999).*

Formal education tends to focus on 'vertical' learning, the accumulation of knowledge. In the workplace, 'horizontal' learning, taking what you know to make sense of the situations you encounter or adapting what you can already do to fit an unexpected presentation is just as important. Medical students and trainees move rapidly from one workplace to another and need to identify and respond to the nuanced differences between one setting or team and another. For example, all doctors routinely take a history from their patients, but there are significant differences in approach across specialties and settings. Clinical teachers can help this process by making expectations explicit (e.g. preferred styles of dress, ways of addressing colleagues and patients, format for writing in notes or constructing letters).

Horizontal learning also needs to help learners activate their formal learning (gained in the classroom) to make sense of clinical encounters. Viewing teaching as a dialogue (rather than a monologue) and using appropriate questioning strategies is particularly effective. Socratic questions can be used to explore what learners know and help them make connections to what they see. Heuristic-type questions, designed to promote the student's own self-directed learning, are also important.

Learning through talking

Social learning theorists suggest that 'talk' is a central part of practice. Learners need to 'learn to talk their way into expertise' rather than just learn from the talk of an expert (Lave and Wenger, 2003).

Many aspects of medical practice are unseen, taking place in the minds of practitioners, engaged in an internal dialogue based around differential diagnosis, clinical reasoning, management planning and exploring prognosis. Clinical teachers need to find ways to make their thinking accessible to the trainee and access the trainee's thinking as a way of ensuring he/she is on track. Strategies include:

'Thinking aloud'

Narratives can be provided as we teach a skill or procedure, or along the lines of 'what I am struggling with here is…' or 'I am weighing up the options of x *vs* y because…'.

Trainee talk

Many clinical teachers have set ways they like trainees to present patients, reflecting ways in which thoughts are organized in order to formulate a diagnosis or management plan. By being clear with trainees that this talking prompts a way of thinking, you are labelling it as a teaching strategy rather than a personal quirk and helping learners to gain insight into how medicine is practised in specific contexts. These ways of talking about patients reveal cultural practices. For example, the way a patient is presented in surgery is different from medicine which is different from psychiatry.

Case-based discussion

This is designed to explore the thinking behind practice. It provides an opportunity for learners to make their thinking explicit and develop ideas. Clinical teachers can make the most of these opportunities by using questions that require the trainee to provide a rationale for decision-making. For example, 'you decided to admit this patient, can you tell me more about the factors that you took into account... how might you justify sending this same patient home... who else in the team did you involve or could you involve in that decision-making process?'

Conclusions

With a reduction in the length of training programmes, a shorter working week, and reduced in-patient exposure workplace-based learning has never been more important. By drawing upon contemporary views on workplace-based learning, clinicians can build upon the sound traditions of apprenticeship and value the workplace as a key site for medical learning and practice.

KEY POINTS

- Make sure your workplace is invitational for all students and trainees.
- Make opportunities for learning from everyday work explicit.
- Provide opportunities for learners to be actively involved in all aspects of patient care.
- Value and make use of the expertise of all members of your community, including patients.
- Help trainees to learn from your talk and to learn to talk medicine.

References

Billett S (2002) Toward a workplace pedagogy: guidance, participation and engagement. *Adult Education Quarterly* **53**(1): 27–43

Billett S (2004) Workplace participatory practices: conceptualising workplaces as learning environments. *Journal of Workplace Learning* **16**(6): 312–24

Bleakley A (2002) Pre-registration house officers and ward based learning: a new apprenticeship model. *Med Educ* **36**: 9–15

Bleakley A (2006) Broadening conceptions of learning in medical education: the message from team-working. *Med Educ* **40**(2): 150–7

Griffiths T, Guile D (1999) Pedagogy in workbased contexts. In: Mortimore P, ed. *Understanding Pedagogy and it's impact on learning*. Sage, London: 155–74

Kolb D (1984) *Experiential Learning*. Prentice Hall, Englewood Cliffs, NJ

Lave J, Wenger E (2003) *Situated Learning: Legitimate Peripheral Participation*. Cambridge University Press, Cambridge

Swanwick T (2005) Informal learning in postgraduate medical education: from cognitivism to 'culturism'. *Med Educ* **39**(8): 859–65

Wenger E (1998) *Communities of Practice: Learning, Meaning and Identity*. Cambridge University Press, Cambridge

CHAPTER 8

Improve your lecturing

Sam Held and Judy McKimm

Lecturing remains the mainstay of many university courses and conference programmes and when done well it can be an extremely effective large group teaching technique.

This chapter introduces teaching large groups through lecturing, considers how lecturing can be planned and structured, explores techniques teachers can use to maximize learning and suggests how to avoid common pitfalls. It also considers ways to ensure that the learning environment is conducive to learning.

What is lecturing?

Lecture: 15th century from Latin lectus past participle of legere – to read a discourse given to an audience or class for instruction. The origin of the lecture is thought to pre-date the printing press by centuries. Books were scarce and valuable, making the lecturer the gatekeeper of knowledge, which the student had to commit to memory (Brown, 2002). Lecturing is still a widely used teaching method in higher education, particularly in relation to conveying information to large numbers of students. Many of the principles underpinning a good lecture also underpin a good conference presentation.

Why lecture?

Lectures are generally used to teach new knowledge and skills, promote reflection and stimulate further learning. If the context is appropriate and they are done well, lectures are an effective means of teaching. The main benefits of lectures are that they:

- Are an effective way of providing information not easily available from other sources
- Are cost effective for transmitting factual information to a large audience
- Provide background information and ideas, basic concepts and methods, to be developed later in small group activities or individual study
- Can highlight similarities and differences between key concepts
- Can usefully demonstrate processes (Bligh, 2000).
- However, lectures also have some disadvantages:
- The audience is usually passive and may therefore be unengaged
- Note-taking often crowds out time to reflect, question or analyse
- They may be ineffective at changing attitudes or encouraging higher-order thinking
- Lecturing reproduces a power differential where the lecturer is the gatekeeper of knowledge and the audience receives whatever is chosen to be conveyed
- Lectures are not suitable for a wide diversity of ability.
- When to lecture?
- There are numerous sound reasons for choosing to lecture, among them (starting with the most pragmatic):
- When there is no alternative because of the size of group or venue
- When the programme stipulates it
- When part of the purpose is to set guidelines for assignments or exams
- When the aim is to illustrate process and/or problem-solving strategies
- When you want to model academic practice you wish to encourage
- When you are invited!

A good lecture at the right time facilitates learning of the key principles of the subject and, building on previous learning, fits coherently into an overall programme of instruction. One hopes that the lecture may also stimulate further thought.

We often assume that lecturing is the only way to teach a large group, and equally rule out the possibility of lecturing to a small group, but neither is always the case. There are various effective methods of teaching large groups, and a skilled lecturer can also adapt to accommodate smaller groups. Lecturing is often seen as the main method for enabling large groups to learn effectively, but small group techniques can be used effectively in contexts where the lecture might seem to be the default choice. *Table 8.1* considers different group sizes in relation to the role of the teacher and considers activities or materials that might be helpful in each context.

Table 8.1 Teaching different sizes of group

Group size	Examples	Role of teacher or instructor
Large groups	Conventional lectures and expositions, workshops, conferences, lab classes, distance and online learning, conferencing, teleconferencing	Traditional role: controller of the process. Some interaction is possible but this requires careful planning
Small group learning	Tutorials, seminars, group exercises and projects, games and simulations, role play, self-help groups, discussions	Organiser and facilitator
Individualised	Directed study (reading books, handouts, discovery learning instruction learning), open learning, distance learning, and guide-programmed learning, mediated self-instruction, computer/web-based learning, e-learning, one to one, work shadowing, mentoring	Producer or manager of learning resources, tutor, supervisor

Adapted from Ellington and Race (1993)

What makes a good lecturer?

There is some mythology about lecturing, the most persistent being that some people have an extraordinary flair for lecturing, and if you are not among the fortunate few, then the best you can hope for is to get through your material with little drama and few problems. Clearly some people are more comfortable presenting to large groups than others, but lectures are primarily to facilitate learning, not for entertainment. A performance might be more relevant at a conference to engage your audience and make your talk memorable. Effective lecturing is more about skill than charisma although some techniques will make your lectures more enjoyable for the audience.

The main characteristics of a good lecturer are that he/she:

- Presents material in a clear and logical sequence
- Makes it accessible, intelligible and meaningful
- Covers the subject matter adequately
- Is constructive and helpful in criticism
- Demonstrates an expert (and authoritarian) knowledge in the subject
- Paces the lecture appropriately
- Is concise

- Illustrates practical applications of the theory presented
- Shows enthusiasm for the subject
- Generates curiosity early in the lecture.

Another myth about lecturing is that as long as the material is interesting it will attract and hold the audience's attention. As the lecturer you may think it fascinating, but even highly motivated learners need more than just interesting material. An effective lecture should present information that cannot be learned from simply reading up on the lecture subject, and use good teaching techniques.

How to make your lecture a success

Consider the purpose

First ask yourself what the purpose of the lecture is and what your audience is there for. Is the main purpose of the lecture to motivate the learners to appreciate the importance of the subject material, or to transmit a body of information not readily attainable elsewhere; to teach important concepts and principles, or is it a reference point in the course, consolidating learning from other contexts or revision for an assessment. If there is more than one purpose, the lecture should deal with them sequentially not concurrently. Adequate time should be allowed for each component.

Define your aims and outcomes

Defining learning outcomes is essential before preparing a lecture. What do you want people to learn? What key concepts are to be addressed? What essential knowledge and understanding should participants leave the lecture with?

Plan a coherent structure

Attention to these questions helps to define structure, content and teaching methods. If, for example, your aim is to present new knowledge and concepts, then the 'classic' lecture structure might be the first choice (*Figure 8.1*). However, if the aim is to present a number of different approaches to a particular problem the method and structure could be quite different (*Figure 8.2*).

The technique in *Figure 8.2* is suited to a lecture in which the purpose is to get students or trainees to learn and model approaches to problem-

Figure 8.1. 'Classic' lecture structure. From Cantillon (2003).

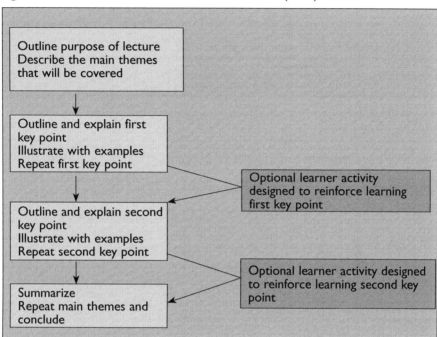

Figure 8.2. 'Problem-oriented' approach. From Cantillon (2003).

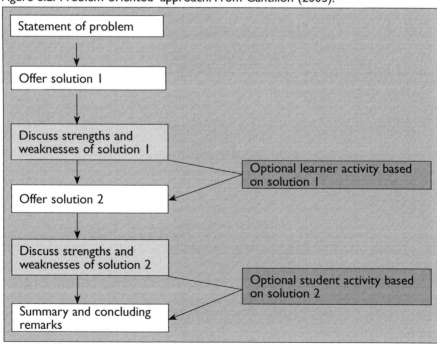

solving. The opening statement of the problem may take the form of a clinical situation or case history, then learners are asked to consider possible solutions. This method is good for encouraging audience participation.

A coherent structure will usually ensure greater retention of the material by the audience. It must provide a logical progression of material and systematically develop your main points: from general principles to specifics, building up the parts into the whole, describing a problem and outlining a solution.

Signal stages of your structure by using the following:

- Signposts – statements that indicate structure and direction (e.g. 'I want to deal briefly with...' 'First, I will...' 'Next, we shall look into ...')
- Frames – statements that signal the beginning and the end of a section (e.g. 'So that ends...' 'And now, let us look at...'). Framing statements are vital in complex explanations that involve topics and sub-topics
- Foci – emphasize key points through repetition and highlighting statements (e.g. 'So the main point is...', 'The key issue is...', 'This brings us to the crucial factor...')
- Links – use explicit statements to link one part of an explanation to another (e.g. 'But while this may be the solution, it may lead to complications')
- Summaries – remind the students of the essential points and link themes which may have been separately discussed. Summarizing provides an opportunity to compare and contrast, point out similarities and differences (adapted from Pan, 2008).

Apply the 'rule of threes'

In lecturing, as in speech-making, people like things to be presented in threes. From the basic trio of beginning, middle and end, to breaking the middle into three clear segments, to the end consisting of summary, check understanding and close, things seem to work best in threes.

Conveniently, concentration tails off to a low point in about 15–20 minutes, but returns after a short break or change of activity. Many lectures last around an hour, so this provides three natural divisions to plan for.

Less is more

Russell et al (1984) observed lectures in which 90%, 70% and 50% of the sentences revealed new information and established that students retained the lecture information better the lower the level of new content. The remaining time was filled by restating, reinforcing and relating the material to prior learning. It is not how much is delivered but how much is understood and retained that is most important. The lecturer should not be afraid to cut down on quantity and ensure that learning actually takes place. You might make sure material is covered by providing a handout during the lecture, giving an outline and guiding questions before the lecture or providing background information and further reading through e-learning.

Practice your presentation

There are lots of techniques, hints and tips to help you give a good lecture and consequently enjoy its delivery. Good presentation hinges on being:

- Clear – ensure you can be seen and heard and use simple, explicit language
- Knowledgeable – know your subject, be authoritative
- Interesting – make eye contact, show enthusiasm and establish a relationship with your audience.

Presentation style is important. Your job is not to entertain – but try not to be boring. Use your voice for emphasis, contrast or negation and use key words for impact, e.g. 'vital' rather than 'important'. Everyone in the room should be able to hear you clearly. Avoid speaking in a monotone, using 'fillers' like 'you know' or 'okay' and distracting gestures like fiddling with jewellery.

Get off to a good start

Decide how you intend to start the lecture before you begin speaking. Introduce yourself and describe the lecture's aims, objectives and learning objectives or outcomes. Tell your audience what you are about to do, how you will do it and what you expect from them. The beginning of your lecture should engage, encourage curiosity and create expectations. The first 5 minutes are your 'golden window' to establish a meaningful link with your students. Try not to be predictable.

Keep them with you

Throughout your presentation, summarize the main points covered in each section at the end of each section. Vary the format of the lecture, i.e. give students a break or a change every 10–15 minutes. Involve the audience:

build in small group discussions, or 'turn to your neighbour for 3 minutes and discuss …'. Your audience will also be more engaged if you avoid reading the full text of your lecture, or read from endless lists of PowerPoint bullet points. Engage the audience throughout with humour, stories and real-life examples.

End it well

Lectures should have a planned ending so avoid abrupt stops. It is usual to include a summary of the main points including a recapitulation of the key questions posed and/or answered. End with a 'take home message' with which you would like learners to leave, and keep to time.

Lecture notes

Reading out lecture notes is not advisable but preparing them helps you plan your delivery. Extemporaneous delivery needs a prepared outline to create the impression of spontaneity. Using this style, you will make better eye contact and be likely to use better non-verbal communication. If you use this approach, your lecture notes may be bullet points, slides, a diagram or prompt cards, depending on your style. If you plan to move around the lecture theatre make sure you are happy with using the microphone and remote controls.

Audio-visual aids and handouts

Audio-visual aids, such as PowerPoint slides or video, will not transform a lecture on their own and can be distracting. Audio-visual resources should enhance the lecture and clarify the material. Avoid complicated 'busy' slides, reading from slides and addressing the screen. Always plan for a fallback position just in case the technology fails.

Learners are not always fully prepared and may not have the necessary prior knowledge, learning skills or motivation to follow your lecture. Good handouts can compensate for this without spoon-feeding learners. Appropriate handouts provide:

- An outline to help learners follow the lecture, letting them concentrate on processing the information as they hear it
- Essential diagrams so learners are engaging, not drawing pictures
- Materials that are difficult to obtain elsewhere
- Tasks to encourage reflection
- A supplementary reading list.

How to encourage 'active learning'

Without attention to the processes by which memory functions, a lecturer may overwhelm listeners, providing too much unsituated information free from context and real world connections. To be meaningful, it must be put into memory and later be retrievable. Information is acquired through experiences stored in episodic memory, or through propositional knowledge stored in semantic memory. The learner must be able to make connections with previous knowledge and restructure it in the light of new information. Introducing new information without adequate consolidation or reflection can interfere with memory input and storage and learners fail to commit the information to memory (Bligh, 2000). The lecturer must ensure that learners can engage actively, make connections and restructure previous learning.

Conclusions

For all its antiquity and somewhat dowdy image, the place of the lecture in medical education is assured. This partly relates to convenience, when a course requires that large groups be formally taught large bodies of material, but lecturing can also be an effective way to approach transmitting information and/or approaches to problem-solving.

Like all teaching and learning, lecturing requires its own skill set which can be learned and refined through practice and reflection. The most important element of an effective lecture is that it should be a meaningful engagement for the audience and speakers alike, providing relevant learning that cannot readily be accessed by other means and ensuring that learners leave the lecture theatre or classroom better informed (or at least more challenged) than when they entered.

KEY POINTS

- Lecturing is an effective large group teaching technique.

- Lectures need to be well planned and structured.

- Lectures are not simply about delivering large amounts of information to a passive audience.

- Learners will learn more if you break up the lecture with signposts, activities and changes of pace.

- Appropriate use of handouts, audiovisual materials and clinical illustrations will enhance your lectures.

References

Bligh D (2000) *What's the Use of Lectures?* Jossey Bass, San Francisco

Brown S (2002) *Lecturing: a Practical Guide*. Routlege, London

Cantillon P (2003) Teaching large groups. In: Cantillon P, Hutchinson L, Wood D, eds. *BMJ ABC of Learning and Teaching in Medicine*. BMJ Publishing Group, London: 15–18

Ellington H, Race P (1993) *Producing Teaching Materials: a Handbook for Teachers and Trainers*. Kogan Page, London

Pan D (2008) Lectures: a good lecture - the basics. In: *Learning to Teach, Teaching to Learn: A handbook for NUS Teachers*. 5th edn. www.cdtl.nus.edu.sg/handbook/lecture/basics.htm (accessed 12 June 2009)

Russell IJ, Hendricson WD, Herbert RJ (1984) Effects of lecture information density on medical student achievement. *J Med Educ* **59:** 881–9

CHAPTER 9

Small group teaching

Judy McKimm and Clare Morris

Small group teaching is effective in encouraging student engagement and discussion. Clinical teachers can use small group teaching techniques to facilitate learning in a range of settings.

This chapter introduces the topic of small group teaching: how small group teaching can be planned and structured and some of the techniques teachers can use to facilitate group and individual learning. It considers strategies for preventing difficult situations in groups and ensuring an appropriate learning environment.

What is a 'small group'?

What characterizes a 'small group' is not so much its size but the teaching and learning context and the way in which the teacher works with and facilitates the learning process. A typical small group is around eight to twelve learners facilitated by a teacher, but in clinical settings groups may comprise a pair of students or trainees working with a health-care team whereas other small groups may comprise 25 or 30 people. Small sub-groups can also operate within a much larger setting such as a lecture, workshop or conference. The size of the group places limitations on the tasks and functions that it might be expected to perform. *Table 9.1* indicates some of the constraints and positive functions relating to group size. Understanding the way in which the size of a group impacts on function is useful if you plan to break up groups into sub-groups or if there are only a small number of learners.

Small group teaching provides opportunities for learning that are difficult to establish in large group settings, although it can be more demanding of staff, space and time. Small group teaching pays attention to group processes as well as to achievement of tasks.

The role of the teacher

There are three main activities that small group teachers have to manage simultaneously:

- Managing the group
- Managing activities
- Managing the learning.

The role of the teacher is typically that of facilitator of learning: leading discussions, asking open-ended questions, guiding process and task, and enabling active participation of learners and engagement with ideas.

Table 9.1. Group size and dynamics		
Size	**Task functions**	**Affective functions**
Individuals	Personal reflection Generating personal data	Personal focus increases 'safety', personal focus means positive start, brings a sense of belonging to and ownership
Twos or threes	Generating data, checking out data, sharing interpretations, good for basic communication skills practice (e.g. listening, questioning, clarifying), good sizes for cooperative working	Builds sense of safety, builds sense of confidence by active involvement (self belief), lays foundation for sharing and cooperating in bigger group, reticent members can still take part
Four to ten	Generating ideas, criticizing ideas, usually sufficient numbers to enable allocation of roles and responsibilities, therefore wide range of work can be tackled (e.g. project work, problem-based learning, syndicate exercises)	Decreasing safety for reticent members, at lower end of the range still difficult for members to 'hide', this risk increases with size, strong can still enthuse the weak, size of group still small enough to avoid splintering, sufficient resources to enable creative support
More than ten	Holding on to a task focus becomes difficult, size hinders discussion but workshop activities possible, e.g. using purposeful sub-groups to address some of the issues	Difficulties in maintaining supportive climate, 'hiding' becomes common, 'dominance' temptation and leadership struggles a risk, divisive possibilities with spontaneous splintering into sub-groups

However, teachers need to be able to adopt a range of roles to respond to the ways small groups function and behave. Richmond (1984) sets out five key roles of the teacher in terms of the 'strategic interventions' required to maintain the group as a functional unit:

1. Start and finish group work – keeping to time, ensuring outcomes and tasks are explained and that the activities draw to a close with learning needs being achieved
2. Maintain the flow of content – ensuring learning follows in a logical sequence and providing stimulus materials and questions
3. Manage group dynamics
4. Facilitate goal achievement – of the wider curriculum, of the session and those identified by the learners themselves
5. Manage group environment – both physical and psychological.

Group dynamics

Understanding the internal dynamics of the group and how to manage different learners makes group working more effective. One useful way of thinking about the ways in which groups develop over time is Tuckman's (1965) framework (*Figure 9.1*):

Forming – when a group comes together for the first time. Teachers can help by facilitating introductions, using ice breaking tasks, explaining the tasks and purpose of the group

Norming – the group begins to share ideas, thought and beliefs and to develop shared norms (group rules). The teacher can help by clarifying

Figure 9.1. Tuckman's model of group process.

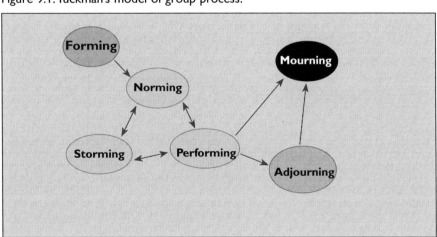

ideas and ground rules, encouraging more reticent people to participate and moving the group towards its purpose

Storming – the group is actively trying to carry out a task and there may be conflict between one or more group members as the group sorts itself out and becomes more functional. The teacher can help by clarifying and reflecting ideas, smoothing over and moderating conflicts and acting as a go-between between members

Performing – the group focuses on the activity and starts to work together as a team to perform the set tasks. The teacher's role is to keep the group focussed and to encourage and facilitate as necessary.

Closure is important, the final stages include 'adjourning' (e.g after each session) or, in the case of a group that has successfully worked together, 'mourning'.

Groups can loop back into the norming or storming stages, especially if there are some personality clashes in the group or difficulties with learning or understanding the tasks. The tutor needs to keep an eye on process and well as task or outputs and intervene if necessary: 'making the right sorts of nudges and interventions ... by using more structure and less intervention in the group process' (Jacques, 2003).

Structuring small group teaching

Small group sessions work well if there is a mix of activities and timings, so that people can work individually, in different-sized groups and with and without teachers. A rule of thumb is that effective concentration on one activity (such as listening to someone talk) lasts around 10 minutes without a break or change of pace. Including breaks and different activities keeps the session flowing, and concentration and learning occurring. However, it is equally important to allow time for groups to bond and work together on shared tasks and not to keep switching people round just for the sake of it.

Types of sessions

Small group teaching takes many forms including seminars, tutorials, workshops, journal clubs, action learning sets, problem-based learning groups and case presentations (www.faculty.londondeanery.ac.uk/e-learning/ small-group-teaching describes different events). When planning small group teaching, think about the learners who will be involved, the resources available (teachers, facilitators, 'experts', patients, rooms, equipment), the learners' needs and the learning outcomes that are to be achieved.

Small group teaching can be built around:
- Topics or themes, e.g. evidence-based practice, asthma, chronic lung conditions
- Clinical cases (actual patients or case notes), e.g. Mrs X presents …with ….
- Clinical or community-based problems, e.g. problem-based learning, a child with a wheeze
- Situations, e.g. critical incident or significant event analysis
- Tasks or skills, e.g. X-ray meetings, clinical audit, examination of cardio-vascular system.

Planning and preparation

Small group teaching provides opportunities for in-depth discussion, reflection and consolidation of learning. Planning can be enhanced by thinking about both 'teacher' and 'learner' activity. For example, a lesson plan may be very detailed or a simple outline, identifying key aims and outcomes, structure and timing of activities to enhance learning, content and key topics and learning resources (see Chapter 3).

Jacques defines three steps (*Figure 9.2*) in planning the structure of a small discussion group.

Figure 9.2. Planning the structure of a small discussion group. From Jacques (2003).

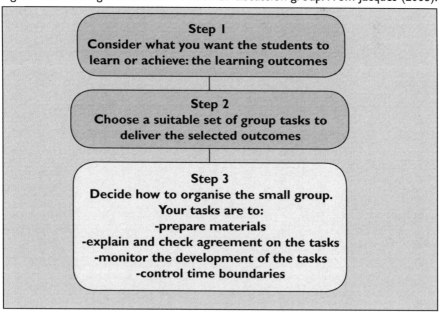

Figure 9.3. Setting out the room. T = teacher.

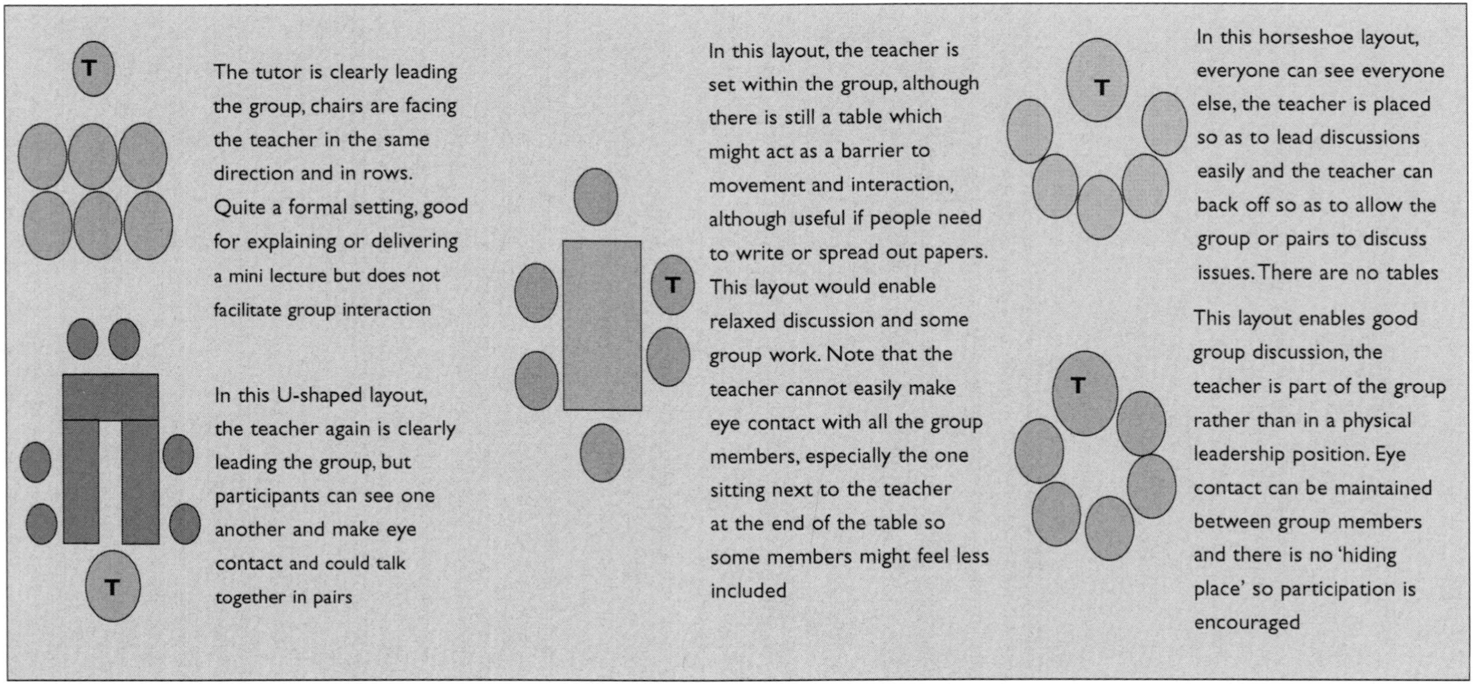

The tutor is clearly leading the group, chairs are facing the teacher in the same direction and in rows. Quite a formal setting, good for explaining or delivering a mini lecture but does not facilitate group interaction

In this U-shaped layout, the teacher again is clearly leading the group, but participants can see one another and make eye contact and could talk together in pairs

In this layout, the teacher is set within the group, although there is still a table which might act as a barrier to movement and interaction, although useful if people need to write or spread out papers. This layout would enable relaxed discussion and some group work. Note that the teacher cannot easily make eye contact with all the group members, especially the one sitting next to the teacher at the end of the table so some members might feel less included

In this horseshoe layout, everyone can see everyone else, the teacher is placed so as to lead discussions easily and the teacher can back off so as to allow the group or pairs to discuss issues. There are no tables

This layout enables good group discussion, the teacher is part of the group rather than in a physical leadership position. Eye contact can be maintained between group members and there is no 'hiding place' so participation is encouraged

Practical arrangements

The physical environment is particularly important in small group work. Paying attention to basic physiological needs such as comfort, noise levels, and lighting can help foster a positive learning environment (Maslow, 1943). The layout of the room clearly signals expectations about the ways in which learners should interact with the teacher and each other. *Figure 9.3* shows examples of room layouts for different activities.

For larger groups, tables can be set out in 'cafeteria' or 'cabaret' style, each seating five or six people, with the teacher and equipment at the front of the room. This enables participants to talk and work in small groups and move around easily. The facilitator can circulate when the groups are working.

Starting the session

Teachers need to establish an appropriate micro-culture within the group, including the physical environment, the psychological climate, the interactions between the teacher and the groups and between the individual group members. The main task for the teacher at the start of the session is to facilitate forming and norming through:

- Creating a positive and welcoming learning environment
- Outlining expectations and exploring group learning needs
- Negotiating and setting ground rules
- Identifying, agreeing and assigning roles and responsibilities
- Facilitating participation and enabling communication through setting appropriate tasks.

Use people's names, plan for introductions and set out the room to facilitate learning and your planned activities. 'Ice-breaker' activities can provide a fun, non-threatening start to group sessions. It usually helps to establish ground rules such as starting and finishing on time, not interrupting, participating, saying when you don't understand, switching off mobile phones, treating others' contributions with respect and maintaining confidentiality.

Teaching strategies

The role of the teacher can be more or less directive with particular activities or session varying from being more teacher- or learner-centred. Strategies that foster interaction between learners include:

- Buzz groups: for quick sharing of ideas then feedback to whole group

- Soap box debates: encouraging learners to adopt a given position on an issue
- Role rehearsal: in triads with an observer to rehearse consultation skills
- Posters: flipcharts and pens can be use to create posters on a key topic
- Task groups: breakout activities to consolidate or develop ideas, e.g. write a patient information leaflet on...

Using different types of questioning to shift the learning and participation focus facilitates discussions and promotes interactions (Jacques, 2000) (*Figures 9.4* and *9.5*).

Figure 9.4. Questioning and facilitation techniques.
a. The teacher (T) is in a more didactic role with interactions being between the teacher and individual learners.
b. Participation is much more active with interactions between participants as well as the teacher.

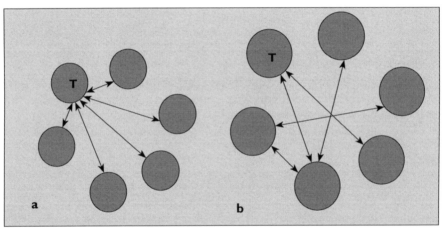

Figure 9.5. Learner and tutor-centred learning. Adapted from Jacques (2000)

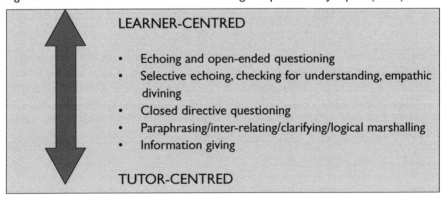

Question strategies

Different question strategies can be used to elicit different responses, stimulate deeper thinking and reflection and promote critical thinking and discussion such as:

Evidence

How do you know that? What evidence is there to support that position?

Clarification

Can you put that another way? Can you give me an example? Can you explain that term?

Explanation

Why might that be the case? How would we know that? Who might be responsible for?

Linking and extending

Is there any connection between what you have just said and what Y said earlier? How does this idea support or challenge what we explored earlier in the session?

Hypothetical

What might happen if? What would be the potential benefits of X?

Cause and effect

How is this response related to management? What is or isn't drug X suitable in this condition? What would happen if we increased or decreased X?

Summary and synthesis

What remains unsolved or uncertain? What else do we need to know or do to understand this better or be better prepared? (adapted from Brookfield, 2006).

Handling problems or difficult situations

> *'If you haven't got problems in your group, then something is wrong.'*
> *(Jacques, 2000)*

Jacques (2003) suggests that common problems associated with leading effective small groups include:
- Teachers lecturing rather than conducting a dialogue
- Teachers talking too much
- Students' reluctance to engage in discussion with one another but only responding to the tutor's questions
- Students not preparing
- Individual students dominating or blocking discussion
- Students wanting to be given solutions to problems rather than discuss them.

One strategy is to let the group sort out its own problems which is effective in the long term and worthwhile if a group is to remain together for some time. However, if the group is very new or working together for a very short time (e.g. a workshop) or has a complex and essential task to perform with a short deadline, then tutor intervention will help keep the group task focussed, for example:
- The persistent talker – summarize points and divert the discussion to others, give them specific tasks, break up the group so that the talker cannot monopolise discussions, or be direct and indicate time pressures
- Quiet people – give time to respond, protect from teasing, divide the group into pairs on a task to increase confidence or positively reinforce any contribution
- Negative attitude – these people may like to talk but have a negative attitude that can affect others. Ask for specific examples, invite the group to think of the positive or defuse lengthy debates.

Closing the session

The final task of the facilitator is to close and conclude the session. Here it is important to leave time to wrap up activities and review the learning outcomes, making sure that you also attend to concluding group processes as well as task functions. It is helpful to link the session to the learners' next steps and ensure any follow-up activities are clear.

Conclusions

Small group techniques are useful to encourage learners' engagement with a topic and with other group members. They can be used in a range of settings from the bedside or clinic to the lecture theatre as well as in more typical classroom settings. The teacher's role as facilitator of learning is a vital component in ensuring effective group working and engagement of all members in task and process.

KEY POINTS

- Small group techniques can be used in a range of settings.
- Plan the session and activities according to the size of group and venue.
- Include a range of activities to encourage active learning and participation.
- Your role in the group learning process may include group leader, facilitator or observer.
- It is important to pay attention to group dynamics to ensure effective group process as well as achievement of tasks.

References

Brookfield S (2006) Discussion as a way of teaching. At: http://stephenbrookfield.com/pdf_files/Discussion_Materials.pdf (accessed 26 February 2008)

Jacques D (2000) The tutors' job. In: Jacques D, ed. *Learning in Groups*. 3rd edn. Kogan Page, London: 155–80

Jacques D (2003) Teaching small groups. In: Cantillon P, Hutchinson L, Wood D, eds. *BMJ ABC of Learning and Teaching in Medicine*. BMJ Publishing Group, London: 19–21

Maslow AH (1943) A theory of human motivation. *Psychol Rev* **50**: 370–96

McCrorie P (2006) *Teaching and leading small groups*. ASME UME series. ASME, Edinburgh

Richmond DE (1984) Improving the effectiveness of small-group learning with strategic intervention. *Med Teach* **6***:* 138–45

Tuckman BW (1965) Developmental sequence in small groups. *Psychol Bull* **63**: 384–99

CHAPTER 10

Involving patients in clinical teaching

Judy McKimm

The interdependent relationship between the clinical teacher, the learner and the patient is a vital part of clinical education. Changing health services and patient expectations have stimulated the need for teachers to consider patients' rights and needs as active participants and partners in clinical teaching.

This chapter introduces the scope, principles and practice of patient involvement in clinical education and considers the application of best practice in patient involvement to the education and training of health professionals. It also examines ethical and practical questions about using real patients and balancing the needs of students and patients in teaching situations.

What is meant by patient involvement?

Involving people in health care has been an important aspect of successive UK government policies since the late 20th century, and it is now an underlying principle of the 'patient-led NHS'. It is a statutory requirement that 'patient and public involvement should be part of everyday practice in the NHS' (Department of Health, 2009); this inevitably includes the training and education of health professionals (General Medical Council, 2009; Morgan and Jones, 2009).

Patient involvement in health care generally clusters around two areas:
1. Active involvement in the health care being given, rather than being a passive recipient of expert advice and treatment
2. Involvement in the development of healthcare services representing their own or the general patient view in decision-making structures.

The patient has always been at the core of medical learning but often as convenient 'teaching material'. There is a need to move the relationship between doctor, learner and patient towards patient-centred learning, where patients are partners in the education process (British Medical Association, 2008). Gordon et al (2000) suggest that patient involvement in clinical teaching can occur in many forms and throughout the whole curriculum cycle: taking an active role in bedside teaching, planning and development of teaching and workplace-based learning sessions and activities.

Why involve patients in clinical teaching?

'For the junior student in medicine and surgery, it is a safe rule to have no teaching without a patient for a text, and the best teaching is that taught by the patient himself' (Osler, 1905).

There are many advantages to involving patients in teaching which Doshi and Brown (2005) list as:

- Learning in context
- Opportunities for role modeling
- Teaching transferable skills
- Increased learner motivation
- Increased professional thinking
- Integration of clinical skills, communication skills, problem solving, decision making and ethical challenges.

However, disadvantages include:

- Its ad-hoc nature
- The decline in availability of patients or clinical cases
- It cannot cover the whole curriculum
- Variations in supervision and delivery
- Conflicting pressures between teaching and service delivery.

Students and trainees express significant benefits of learning with and from patients. Although simulation and other learning methods offer opportunities to practice procedures they only prepare learners for working with patients and are no substitute for learning to practice medicine independently with patients. Learners value working with patients in the context of structured learning events, supported and supervised by more senior clinicians. To develop effective clinical reasoning, learners need to see a wide range of cases in varying contexts (Eva, 2005) but they also need support in making sense of what they see, through discussion with and challenge from clinical teachers.

Which patients should be involved, where and how?

Spencer et al (2000) reviewed the role of the patient in teaching and learning and devised a framework to assist clinical educators in working with patients in any given context. The 'Cambridge framework' is based around checklists identifying Who? How? What? and Where?

Who?

Which patients to involve depends on a number of interconnected factors. These include:
- Presenting clinical problems
- Socioeconomic status, ethnicity, background, culture, experience and expectations of each patient, his/her family and carers
- Age, gender, sexual orientation
- Emotional and intellectual capacity.

While research suggests that the majority of patients benefit from being involved in teaching (Haffling and Håkansson, 2008; Lefroy, 2008), clinical teachers need to decide on the appropriateness of involving patients in teaching after consultation with patients and carers.

How?

Considering 'the how' enables teachers to select the type of interactions that may be most relevant to achieve different learning outcomes for learners (*Figure 10.1*).

Figure 10.1. The 'how' of clinical teaching with patients.
Adapted from Spencer et al (2000).

Brief contact or prolonged contact
Passive role or active role
Time limited or time committed
Trained or untrained
Inexperienced ('novice') or experienced ('expert')
Planned encounter or unplanned encounter
Simulated situation or real situation
'Questioning' or 'informing'
Known patient or unknown patient
Focused learning or holistic learning
Tutor involved or tutor not involved

Where?

The 'where' includes a choice of settings and professional contexts such as:

- 'Real environment' and 'simulated environment' – as training wards and simulation centres are increasingly being used in training health professionals
- 'Uni-professional' or 'multiprofessional' settings – clinical situations in which doctors alone are learning with patient or where a range of professionals are learning and working (*Figure 10.2*).

The location of the encounter (e.g. patients' homes, GP practice, intensive care unit) has a huge impact on the patients' and learners' experiences and the learning opportunities available. The location affects the learning that can take place while the patient is present, the preparatory and follow up learning, and the roles and expectations of teacher, patient and learner (Spencer and McKimm, 2010).

What?

Considering the sort of learning (the content) or clinical problems that the trainee might encounter when working with different patients can help to tease out what specifically the learner is gaining from listening to and examining the patient (*Figure 10.3*).

This also helps clinical teachers assess what can be expected of the learning situation with different patients and in different contexts and what the likely impact on or value is, both for patients and learners, of involving the patient in a given situation.

Figure 10.2. The 'where' of clinical teaching with patients.
Adapted from Spencer et al (2000).

Figure 10.3. The 'what' of clinical teaching with patients.
Adapted from Spencer et al (2000).

'Our place' or 'your place'
Community or hospital
'My culture' or 'your culture'
'My clothes' or 'your clothes'
Service setting or educational setting

Undifferentiated problem or defined problem
Straightforward or challenging
High impact or low impact
General or specific
Clinical science or basic science
Minor or major
Simple skills or complex skills
'Revealed' attitudes or 'hidden' attitudes
Particular focus or generic approach

What sort of patient?

Real patients in real clinical areas

One of the real benefits to learners in working with real patients in the clinical context is that they can consolidate and synthesize their learning from a range of sources.

Whenever clinical teaching occurs with real patients, patients are usually the most vulnerable of the three parties involved. Most patients still find clinical teaching extremely rewarding, often commenting that they feel students 'have to learn'. The patient's contribution to teaching should always be respected and he/she should know that, should he/she wish to withdraw, it will not affect treatment and care. Patients must be made explicitly aware that they are in a teaching environment, that learners may be present and sometimes helping to provide their care. This allows the patient to raise any anxieties. The patient needs to be kept informed, mutual agreement needs to be reached about every session, and patient privacy and dignity must always be maintained. Explain to the patient the number and level of the learners who may be present, what the patient might be expected to do and clarify the patient's proposed role. Verbal agreement should be obtained and documented.

While involving real patients in teaching in clinical areas is often opportunistic (based on who is on the ward or attending the clinic or surgery), the same steps must be taken in all cases.

Expert patients

These are 'real' patients who are trained to deliver teaching sessions acting as both patient and teacher. The idea of the expert patient is part of the wider patient involvement agenda: it was targeted at patients with chronic conditions to help them 'become key decision-makers in their own care' (Hardy, 2004). In medical education, the expert patient role is that of a patient who agrees to participate in teaching and learning. He/she is seen as an 'expert' in his/her own condition and is often briefed or trained so as to facilitate student or trainee learning.

Patient educators have the benefits of being:

- Motivated individuals with an interest in medical training
- Real patients with real clinical histories and signs
- Able to give structured feedback to learners and teachers from the patient's perspective, such as the pressure of the hands or the way in which a history was taken.

Expert patients can help overcome educational challenges involving intimate examinations. For example female patient educators are commonly used to teach gynaecological and breast examination. They can also help to free up clinical tutors as, once trained, patient educators need little assistance in running sessions and can also be used in clinical assessments (standardized and objective). Expert patients or patient educators can be drawn from many settings, even those where concerns might be expressed about the potential risk to patients, such as those who are terminally ill or with mental health problems.

Using video and audio

Although clearly not the 'traditional' doctor–patient–student triad, the 'patient voice' can be incorporated into clinical teaching using a whole range of resources including video, case scenarios, sound recordings and e-learning resources. Many of these resources are freely available, including interactive computerized tutorials on topics such as epileptic seizure classification (Farrar et al, 2008) or breaking bad news (Cleland et al, 2007). These resources are helpful when it is inappropriate or difficult for learners to work with real patients, for example tropical medicine, child protection or terminal illness, and enable a more standardized approach to assessment of clinical skills or knowledge.

What do patients think?

Most research into patient views on involvement in teaching emphasizes the positive nature of the encounter, 'even unprepared patients see themselves as contributors to teaching' (Haffling and Håkasson, 2008). Patients often see themselves as experts on their condition and facilitators of learning, particularly in professional skills and attitudes (Stacey and Spencer, 1999). Empowering patients includes providing 'opportunities for communication and input, being asked for their consent; having their feedback valued' (Howe and Anderson, 2003).

Benefits cited by patients include:

- Feelings of altruism and helpfulness
- 'Repaying the system'
- Learning more about their clinical condition or problem
- Being given more time and attention by clinicians – a better service
- Being valued and enhancing self-esteem
- Reassurance of wellbeing ('a good going over') (O'Flynn et al, 1997; Coleman and Murray, 2002; Howe and Anderson, 2003).

Factors that cause patients to feel reluctant to participate in clinical teaching include:

- Embarrassment about emotional problems or intimate examinations
- Gender or cultural factors, for example male students practising gynaecological procedures (O'Flynn and Rymer, 2002)
- Previous poor experiences with learners
- Relatively large numbers or less experienced learners
- When the consultation or encounter is 'high stakes' (such as birth, being given bad news, a difficult, painful or sensitive examination or procedure)
- Repeated contact with doctors and learners can also reinforce feelings of ill-health, emphasizing the medicalization of health issues (Coleman and Murray, 2002).

Benson et al (2005) also identified that patients perceive differences between what they might accept as the norm in hospital and in general practice, which is seen more as the 'patient's territory'. The Postgraduate Medical Education and Training Board (2008) suggested that medical colleges should involve a greater diversity of patients in education and training, expectations of patients must be clearly indicated, interviews could be filmed to take the pressure off less confident patients and a national bank of case studies could be developed to reflect the UK's diverse population.

Ethical issues

It is not acceptable to simply assume it is okay to involve patients in teaching and learning. Key ethical issues to be considered when involving patients can be summarized as the 'three Cs': consent, choice and confidentiality.

Consent

'A mindset shift needs to occur within the medical profession to enable informed partnership rather than informed consent (patient)' (Postgraduate Medical Education and Training Board, 2008). Medical law and ethics enshrine the principle of informed (patient) consent, particularly relating to medical procedures. However, in teaching and learning, this is often tacit and assumed. Teachers need to remember to inform patients (ideally in writing in advance) that students may be involved in their care. Howe and Anderson (2003) suggest that obtaining consent is 'a continuous process that begins with the first contact the service has with the patient'.

Choice

Trainees need to learn from patients and practice procedures within the 'turbulent here and now of care delivery' (Hardy and Stanton, 2007). Clinical teachers can ensure patient choice through seeking agreement without the learner being present, confirming choice in the presence of learners (Howe and Anderson, 2003) and building in opportunities for patients to say no to specific tasks. Note also that patients may have less personal power and space in an acute setting (Benson et al, 2005).

Confidentiality

Practical steps that help to maintain confidentiality include:
- Providing information so patients understand the boundaries of confidentiality
- Reassuring the patient, involving him/her in discussions
- Finding private spaces to discuss intimate issues
- Remembering that curtains around a bed do not provide privacy
- Discussing confidentiality actively with trainees
- Obtaining permission for the use of any recorded media.

Optimizing the opportunities

'The bedside is the perfect venue for unrehearsed and unexpected triangular interactions between teacher, trainees and patient' (Ramani, 2003). Paradoxically, unrehearsed and unexpected 'moments' work best when prepared for.

Before the session involving patients, think about:
- What preparatory work the trainee needs (e.g. reading, skills laboratory)
- Where the teaching will occur
- Which parts of the session require direct patient contact
- Whether you will be present when the trainee is with the patient
- What role you will take (observer, instructor, demonstrator, questioner)
- Where discussions will take place (do they have to be round the bedside?)
- How to build in opportunities for patient feedback
- How to build in debriefs for learner and patient
- What follow up learning or reading should be carried out.

Janicik and Fletcher (2003) suggest that clinical teachers need to attend to aspects in three domains:

1. Attending to the patient's comfort
2. Focusing on the microskills of teaching, modified for the bedside
3. Attending to group dynamics and giving feedback.

Spencer and McKimm (2010) also suggest that if teachers attend to the ongoing dialogue between learner, teacher and patient (the 'trialogue') the development of both therapeutic and learning alliances between all parties is facilitated. Another structured model for teaching involving patients is shown in *Table 10.1*.

Table 10.1. A model for patient-based teaching	
Shadowing (role modeling)	Trainee shadows a more senior clinician and learns by observation Tip – before the session identify active observation focus or questions that the trainee will specifically look for
Patient-centred	Trainee is allocated patients and follows their progress from start to end of episode of illness Tip – useful to help trainees actively learn patient management and problem solving, needs support through guided reading and discussion from teachers
Reporting back	Trainee assesses the patients and reports back to the trainer Tip – teacher needs to build in identified briefing and debriefing time with a structure and purpose to the feedback
Direct observation	The trainer observes the trainee's performance directly Tip – follow rules of feedback, good for learning clinical skills, take care not to leave the patient as a passive participant in the process, think of how the patient might feed back to the trainee
Videoing interviews	The trainee's interview with a patients is recorded and later viewed with the trainer Tip – needs consent from patient re images, good for learning consultation and communication skills, can be done with a group or single trainee. Take care that the trainee does not over-dwell on minor issues
Case conference	A case is presented by the trainee and discussed by a wider audience Tip – useful for multi-professional learning and inputs, teacher supports trainee re the type of questions that might come up and how to present a case
From Doshi and Brown (2005)	

Conclusions

Involving patients in teaching and learning is a vital element of equipping doctors with the skills, knowledge and behaviours that will enable them to become effective, caring and compassionate practitioners.

Effective involvement of patients in teaching is founded on good clinical care, which can help support or diminish patients' capacity for self-care and autonomy. Real involvement of patients (and carers) in teaching and learning means that they share in the learning process. This can range from active involvement in lesson planning, assessment or leading teaching sessions, to a less active role, but one that nevertheless includes the patient in the learning process as a partner, thus reflecting the shift highlighted by the Postgraduate Medical Education and Training Board (2008): 'every patient should be considered a teacher as well as a patient'.

KEY POINTS

- Consider whether learning objectives can best be achieved involving patients, is it in the patients' best interests or can they be achieved using some other method?
- Consent is about involvement and partnership.
- Introduce questioning before and after the encounter to stimulate learners' awareness of how they can learn from and appreciate the patient's input.
- Plan the session to encourage patient (and carer) participation.
- Actively consider your own involvement in the learning session with patients, in the light of the trainee's experience and competence and the patient's place on his/her health journey.
- Clinical teachers are role models to learners both as a clinician and as a teacher.

References

Benson J, Quince T, Hibble A, Fanshawe T, Emery J (2005) Impact on patients of expanded, general practice based, student teaching: observational and qualitative study. *BMJ* **331**(7508): 89 (doi: 10.1136/bmj.38492.599606.8F)

British Medical Association (2008) *The role of the patient in medical education.* www.bma. org.uk/careers/medical_education/roleofthepatient.jsp (accessed 5 July 2010)

Cleland J, Ford R, Hamilton NM, Nabavian S, Walker K (2007) Breaking bad news: an interactive web-based e-learning package. *Clin Teach* **4**(2): 94–9

Coleman K, Murray E (2002) Patients views and feelings on the community-based teaching of undergraduate medical students: a qualitative study. *Family Practice* **19**(2): 183–8

Department of Health (2009) *Creating a Patient-led NHS. Delivering the NHS Improvement Plan*. Department of Health, London (icn.csip.org.uk/_library/Creating_a_patient-led_NHS.pdf accessed 28 June 2010)

Doshi M, Brown N (2005) Whys and hows of patient-based teaching. *Advances in Psychiatric Treatment* **11**: 223–31

Eva K (2005) What every teacher needs to know about clinical reasoning. *Med Educ* **39**: 98–106

Farrar M, Connolly AM, Lawson J, Burgess A, Lonergan A, Bye AME (2008) Teaching doctors how to diagnose paroxysmal events: a comparison of two educational methods. *Med Educ* **42**: 909–14

General Medical Council (2009) *Tomorrow's Doctors*. General Medical Council, London

Gordon J, Hazlett C, Ten Cate O et al (2000) Strategic planning in medical education: enhancing the learning environment for students in clinical settings. *Med Educ* **34**: 841–50

Haffling A, Håkansson A (2008) Patients consulting with students in general practice: survey of patient's satisfaction and their role in teaching. *Med Teach* **30**: 622–9

Hardy P, Stanton P (2007) Cultivating compassion: seeing Patient Voices. *BMJ* **335**: 184–7

Hardy P (2004) The expert patient programme: a critical review. MSc Lifelong learning, policy and research. www.pilgrimprojects.co.uk/papers/epp_msc.pdf (accessed 27 June 2010)

Howe A, Anderson J (2003) Involving patients in medical education. *BMJ* **327**: 326–8

Janicik RW, Fletcher KE (2003) Teaching at the bedside: a new model. *Med Teach* **25**: 127–30

Lefroy J (2008) Should I ask my patient with cancer to teach students? *Clin Teach* **5**: 138–42

Morgan A, Jones D (2009) Perceptions of service user and carer involvement in healthcare education and impact on students' knowledge and practice: a literature review. *Med Teach* **31**: 82–95

O'Flynn N, Rymer J (2002) Women's attitude to the sex of medical students in a gynaecology clinic: cross-sectional survey. *BMJ* **325**: 683–84

O'Flynn N, Spencer J, Jones R (1997) Consent and confidentiality in teaching general practice: survey of patients' views on presence of students. *BMJ* **315**: 1142

Osler W (1905) The hospital as a college. In: *Aequanimatus and Other Addresses*. HK Lewis, London

Postgraduate Medical Education and Training Board (2008) *Training in Partnership: The Patient Perspective: Shaping the future of postgraduate medical education and training in the UK – the patient perspective.* PMETB, London (www.gmc-uk.org/9_May_2008_Patient_Perspective_Seminar_Report_.pdf_30426823.pdf (accessed 22 July 2010)

Ramani S (2003) Twelve tips to improve bedside teaching. *Med Teach* 25(2): 112–15

Spencer J, McKimm J (2010) Involving patients in clinical education. In: Swanwick T, ed. *Understanding Medical Education.* Wiley Blackwell, London

Spencer J, Blackmore P, Heard S et al (2000) Patient-oriented learning: a review of the role of the patient in the education of medical students. *Med Educ* 34: 851–7

Stacey R, Spencer J (1999) Patients as teachers: a qualitative study of patients' views on their role in a community based undergraduate project. *Med Educ* 33: 688–94

CHAPTER 11

Workplace-based assessment

Tim Swanwick and Nav Chana

This chapter outlines some of the principles underpinning the design of workplace-based assessment and considers some of the tools that have been adopted for use within assessment programmes. The unique challenges of workplace-based assessment are considered, in particular the thorny issue of 'reliability'.

What is workplace-based assessment?

Workplace-based assessment refers to the assessment of what doctors actually do in practice and is predominantly carried out in the workplace itself. Workplace-based assessment in the training context relies on the use of tools for gathering information about aspects of trainees' work which are then used as vehicles for offering direct, timely and relevant feedback. The collection of workplace-based assessment data is learner-led and brought together, usually in a portfolio of evidence, to inform judgments about the trainee's overall progress.

So how does workplace-based assessment fit with traditional forms of testing in medicine?

Miller (1990) provides a useful pyramidal model (*Figure 11.1*) for mapping assessment methods currently available in medical education and illustrates how workplace-based assessment relates to the assessment of clinical competence.

'Knows' forms the base of Miller's pyramid, the entry point in the development of expertise. This tier is best assessed using simple knowledge tests such as multiple choice questions. The next tier up 'knows how' seeks to measure understanding or application of knowledge and is assessed using instruments such as unfolding patient management problems, extended matching or short essay questions. Higher up, objective structured clinical examinations assess at the 'shows how' level where students are required to demonstrate not only knowledge and understanding, but that they can bring together and manipulate relevant knowledge, skills and attitudes in a controlled situation.

Figure 11.1 'Miller's pyramid'. From Miller (1990).

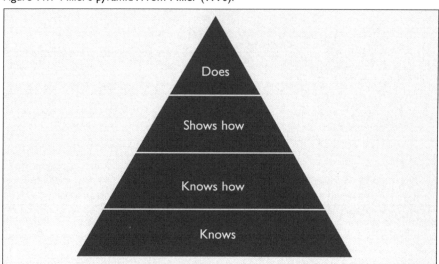

The problem is that what doctors do in controlled assessment situations correlates poorly with their actual performance in professional practice (Rethans et al, 2002). Assessment of competence in a contextual vacuum is all very well but how can we know what happens in the messiness of real professional practice – what the doctor actually 'does'? This is where workplace-based assessment comes into its own.

Is it useful?

The utility, or usefulness, of an assessment has been defined as a product of its reliability, validity, cost-effectiveness, acceptability and educational impact (van der Vleuten, 1996). Utility can be applied to an entire assessment system or to an individual assessment method or component of the system. The concept is important in that no single element should be regarded as predominant. Assessment design then inevitably leads to a trade off between individual elements. Thus, traditional approaches to maximize the reliability or reproducibility of assessments can have a negative educational impact on the learner by reducing the opportunity for meaningful developmental feedback. Workplace-based assessments offer high educational impact but might not be as reliable as other highly structured tests such as multiple choice questions.

Historically, the seductiveness of standardized testing led medical education to rely on externally administered assessments delivered at the end of programmes of training. Workplace-based assessment offers an opportunity to re-evaluate this situation and reintegrate teaching, learning

Figure 11.2 The educational paradigm: integrating teaching, learning and assessment.

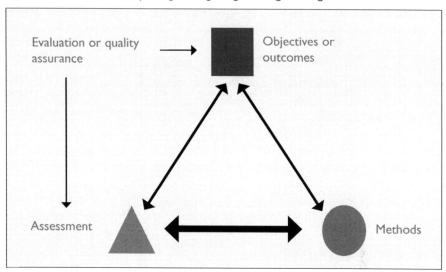

and assessment (*Figure 11.2*), in other words, providing assessment that is 'built in' and not 'bolt on'.

From methods to programmes

Traditional approaches to medical assessment have been founded on the notion that domains of competence (e.g. problem solving, communication skills) are stable and generic. It was considered possible to design tests that assessed these domains separately and reliably leading to a 'one trait, one instrument' approach (Schuwirth and van der Vleuten, 2004). However, there has been a growing realization that competence is specific to particular clinical situations or contexts. In order to overcome this problem, it is vital to sample widely across both the content of the curriculum and the contexts in clinical care is delivered.

Given the complexity of assessing professional competence it is now recognized that assessment should be construed as a programme of activity requiring the acquisition of quantitative and qualitative information from different sources. As a major contribution to such programmes, assessing doctors in their actual working environment offers the opportunity to gather information using a variety of different tools, so building a 'rich picture' of their working practices.

Workplace-based assessments will not replace standardized assessments. There are issues in relation to reliability as a result of inconsistent application of tools by different raters or assessors. There is potential conflict in the role of the trainer who is supervising the learner, but also involved in the assessment process. And there are problems of attribution when routinely collected clinical practice data are assessed. So in order to gain the benefits while mitigating the risks, a number of key issues should be considered in the design and implementation of such assessment programmes.

What to assess?

The areas chosen to assess in workplace-based assessment are usually expressed as a series of competencies. These should be blueprinted against the curriculum and, in the way they are expressed, should encourage learner development. Let us look at those three issues in a little more detail:

Competency-based

Workplace-based assessment is usually competency-based. Despite criticisms of competency-based education as a whole (Talbot, 2004), concerns have usually been voiced where competencies are viewed as narrow, reductionist and overly simplistic. Competencies used for designing workplace-based assessments are best written as holistic statements which are framed as 'a complex structuring of attributes needed for intelligent performance in specific situations' (Gonczi, 1994).

Blueprinted

To ensure that assessments are integrated with the curriculum, competencies chosen for assessment should map directly onto the curriculum to ensure that there is both adequate coverage and widespread sampling. Some aspects of a curriculum will be more efficiently assessed through other means, clinical knowledge being an obvious case in point, however, some will be best assessed in the workplace. Indeed many aspects of professional performance such as team working, leadership and commitment to continuing professional development, are virtually impossible to assess in any other way.

Developmental

As already discussed, workplace-based assessment offers the opportunity to connect teaching, learning and assessment, and the developmental aspect of the assessment should therefore be a key feature. Developmental progressions in the literature, such as the novice to expert progression described by Dreyfus and Dreyfus (1986), may be helpful in constructing a developmental continuum of competence. Such a continuum has the advantage of explicitly illustrating the direction of travel for trainees, rather than merely pointing out the level below which they should not fall. This supports the concept of ongoing evidence collection throughout the training period, but with regular, well-circumscribed staging reviews at which the developmental framework is reviewed and the learner's progress through it judged.

So, workplace-based assessment provides useful formative and developmental feedback but it also has a summative role and informs judgments about overall progress. This raises the tension of potentially mixing formative and summative elements, but it is possible to address this through the careful design of the assessment system. Separating the interpretation of evidence from its elicitation is one way around the problem (Wiliam and Black, 1996). In other words, when it is assessment time, the learner needs to know, and be adequately prepared for it.

How much evidence is enough?

Collecting 'sufficient' evidence is essential in making a judgment about the attainment of competence. As we have seen, sampling widely across a number of clinical and contextual situations is important to overcome the problem of case specificity. In the assessment of 'work' there is no single method that will do it all and a variety of sources of information will be needed. This gives rise to the notion of a 'tool-box' of assessment methods.

In considering individual tools it is worth recognizing that, even unstandardized, they can be made sufficiently reliable, provided the tools are used sensibly and expertly, and enough sampling occurs (van der Vleuten and Schuwirth, 2005). But it is important to remember that the tools themselves only form a small part of an overall assessment programme and attention should focus on the utility of the entire programme of assessment, not just the individual tools themselves.

Confidence in the reproducibility of judgments made on the basis of workplace-based assessment can be improved through triangulation. This involves using a range of different methods to collect evidence using multiple raters over a sustained period of time. Triangulation with other assessments external to the workplace is also important and an overarching assessment strategy for each training programme, in which workplace-based assessment is supported by other test methods – such as those of 'knowledge' and 'skills for clinical method', is essential.

Which methods?

The methods for used for providing feedback and gathering workplace evidence in current use tend to be variations on one of four themes; observations of clinical activities, discussion of clinical cases, analysis of performance data and multi-source feedback.

Observations of clinical activities

Traditionally, clinical skills have been assessed by the 'long case' presentation. The problem of case specificity using this technique, limiting the potential to sample widely, has given rise to the mini-clinical evaluation exercise or mini-CEX (Norcini et al, 1995). This tool has been developed to assess the clinical skills that trainees most often use in real patient encounters. It is based on assessment of multiple complete or partial clinical encounters observed by an educational supervisor or other clinician.

The direct observation of procedural skills (DOPS) is another widely used tool, and one of a number of similar instruments based around the assessment of real-life activities where the focus is on the skill with which the activity was performed. 'The consistent feature is that one or more assessors, who are trained in the assessment of that skill, make a judgment about a real life performance' (Postgraduate Medical Education and Training Board, 2007).

A raft of other observational tools encompassing a wide range of workplace activities are in also current use including the procedure-based assessment of the Intercollegiate Surgical Curriculum, the mini-imaging interpretation exercise of the Royal College of Radiologists and the assessment of teaching of the Royal College of Psychiatrists.

Discussion of clinical cases

The origin of the use of case-based discussion in UK training assessment systems stemmed from their use in the General Medical Council's performance procedures (Southgate et al, 2001) deriving originally from chart-stimulated recall oral assessments used in the USA and Canada. Case-based discussion is one of the evidence gathering tools used in workplace-based assessment in the UK foundation programme and is also being used in specialty training programmes such as in medicine, paediatrics and general practice.

Analysis of performance data

Norcini (2003) describes the basis for making a judgment on clinical performance data as having three potential sources; outcomes, process and volume. Outcomes of care, while being the most desirable measure, are limited by problems of attribution (to the individual), complexity, case mix and numbers. This is a particular problem in the assessment of trainee performance.

The process of care is more directly attributable to the individual doctor but effective processes do not necessarily mirror the best patient outcomes. The use of volumes of activity is premised on the basis that the more of a given activity that a doctor performs, the better their quality of care is likely to be. This basis for judgment is typified by the log books of the craft specialties such as surgery.

Multi-source feedback

The aim of using multi-source feedback to assess doctors in the workplace is to view a person's work from a variety of perspectives. In medical settings, physician colleagues (peers), co-workers and patients can be asked to complete surveys about the doctor. The person being assessed receives feedback based on his/her own aggregate ratings, usually along with average ratings of others being assessed at the same time. There is also a clear opportunity for comparing self-assessment data with those provided by raters.

Multi-source feedback tools can be sub-divided into peer-rating tools, such as the mini-PAT (mini peer-rating assessment tool) used in foundation training, and patient satisfaction questionnaires, a significant number of which are in use in the UK (Chisholm and Askham, 2006).

Portfolios

Workplace-based assessments are usually collected within a structured portfolio. A portfolio comprises a dossier of evidence collected over time, which demonstrates a doctor's education and practice achievements (Wilkinson et al, 2002). There are many portfolio models (Webb et al, 2002) but in essence, if well constructed, a portfolio should chronicle the journey of a learner towards the attainment of professional expertise. A portfolio:

- Aims to serve as the reflective learning log of the learner, available to be shared with his/her educational supervisor

- Demonstrates the learner's progress towards covering the breadth and depth of the curriculum
- Acts as a repository for assessments
- Provides a framework for learning agreements between learners and teachers
- Charts a learner's progression and can help in making career choices and decisions.

The majority of portfolios used in medical education are web-based although with significant differences in structure and design between specialties and stage of training.

Quality assurance

Returning to the concept of utility, workplace-based assessment has huge strengths in the area of validity by virtue of its assessment of real or authentic material. Potentially it may have significant educational impact because of the reconnection of teaching and learning. Acceptability and cost-effectiveness are also potential winners but depend largely on how programmes are implemented. There are, however, significant issues with reliability as understood by traditional psychometric approaches. As Southgate et al (2001) point out, 'establishing the reliability of assessments of performance in the workplace is difficult because they rely on expert judgements of unstandardised material'.

In workplace-based assessment there are several specific threats to reliability:
- Inter-observer variation: the tendency for one observer to mark consistently higher or lower than another
- Intra-observer variation: variation in an observer's performance for no apparent reason (the 'good day/bad day' phenomenon)
- Case specificity: variation in the candidate's performance from one challenge to another, even when they seem to test the same attribute.

In the context of workplace-based assessment it is therefore helpful to reframe reliability as an attempt to maximize 'consistency and comparability'. Baker et al (1992) propose a number of activities that can help to do this, namely:
- Specification of standards, criteria, scoring guides
- Calibration of assessors and moderators
- Moderation of results, particularly those on the borderline
- Training of assessors, with retraining where necessary
- Verification and audit through the collection of assessment data.

It is clear, then, that the implementation of a successful workplace-based assessment programme will require training for assessors, arrangements for calibration, a procedure for the moderation of results and a raft of quality control checks. The more that teachers can be engaged in assessment, for example in selecting methodologies, generating standards and discussing criteria, the more the educational benefits of this powerful form of assessment can be realized.

Conclusions

Workplace-based assessment offers the opportunity to connect teaching, learning and assessment, provides a means for assessment of problematic areas that require evaluation of real performance in practice and is a useful component of an overall assessment programme. In order for its benefits to be realized there needs to be: clarity about what is being assessed through the identification of holistically described professional competencies; attention given to the developmental nature of the assessment; a variety of assessment tools used to gather evidence from multiple clinical contexts using multiple raters; and processes in place by which evidence can be collated, synthesized and judged at regular intervals by an educational supervisor to assess the learner's progress with consistency and comparability across assessment programmes maximized through a robust programme of quality assurance.

KEY POINTS

- Workplace-based assessment is now widespread across all specialities and all stages of training.

- Workplace-based assessment offers the opportunity to connect teaching, learning and assessment.

- Workplace-based assessment has a dual function of offering focussed and timely feedback to trainees as well as providing data to support more long range judgments about trainee progress.

- Workplace-based assessment requires new ways of thinking about reliability based on maximizing consistency and comparability.

References

Baker E, O'Neil H, Linn R (1992) Policy and validity prospects for performance-based assessment. *Am Psychol* 48(12): 1210–18

Chisholm A, Askham J (2006*) What Do You Think of Your Doctor? A review of questionnaires for gathering patients' feedback about their doctor.* Picker Institute, Europe

Dreyfus H, Dreyfus S (1986) *Mind over machine. The Power of Human Intuition Expertise in the Era of the Computer.* Basil Blackwell, Oxford

Gonczi A (1994) Competency based assessment in the professions in Australia. *Assessment in Education 1*(1): 27–44

Miller G (1990) The assessment of clinical skills/competence/performance. *Acad Med* **65**(Suppl): S63–7

Norcini J (2003) ABC of learning and teaching in medicine. Work based assessment. *BMJ* **326***:* 753–5

Norcini J, Blank L, Arnold G, Kimball H (1995) The mini-CEX: a preliminary investigation. *Ann Intern Med* **125***:* 795–9

Postgraduate Medical Education and Training Board (2007) *Developing and Maintaining an Assessment System – a guide to good practice.* Postgraduate Medical Education and Training Board, London

Rethans J, Norcini J, Baron-Maldonado M, Blackmore D, Jolly B, La Duca T (2002) The relationship between competence and performance: implications for assessing practice performance. *Med Educ* **36**: 901–9

Southgate L, Cox J, David T et al (2001) The assessment of poorly performing doctors: the development of the assessment programmes for the General Medical Council's Performance Procedures. *Med Educ* **35**(Suppl 1): 2–8

Schuwirth L, van der Vleuten C (2004) Changing education, changing assessment, changing research. *Med Educ* **38**: 805–12

Talbot M (2004) Monkey see, monkey do: a critique of the competency model in graduate medical education. *Med Educ* **38**: 1–7

van der Vleuten C (1996) The assessment of professional competence: developments, research and practical implications. *Advances in Health Science Education 1:* 41–67

van der Vleuten C, Schuwirth L (2005) Assessing professional competence: from methods to programmes. *Med Educ* **39***:* 309–17

Webb C, Gray M, Jasper M, Miller C, McMullan M, Scholes J (2002) Models of portfolios. *Med Educ* **36**(10): 897–8

Wilkinson TJ, Challis M, Hobma SO, Newble DI, Parboosingh JT, Sibbald JG, Wakeford R (2002) The use of portfolios for assessment of the competence and performance of doctors in practice. *Med Educ* **36***:* 918–24

Wiliam D, Black P (1996) Meanings and consequences: a basis for distinguishing formative and summative functions of assessment? *Br Educ Res J* **22***:* 537–48

CHAPTER 12

Interprofessional learning

Judy McKimm and Dulcie-Jane Brake

Well-functioning multiprofessional teams are key to delivering effective and safe health care. Clinical teachers need to be able to provide opportunities for learners from different health professions to work collaboratively and learn about and from one another.

This chapter provides an introduction to interprofessional learning in relation to medical and health professionals' education. It defines key terms, sets out the policy drivers and provides examples of how interprofessional learning can be implemented in clinical teaching situations. It also considers some of the challenges and barriers to implementing interprofessional learning.

Definitions

Health care is commonly delivered by groups of professionals rather than single professionals. From the patient's perspective, the more closely professions communicate and work together, the more seamless and effective health provision will be. Evidence is growing that if professionals also learn together in an active and structured way, then they are more likely to work collaboratively in practice. *Figure 12.1* explains some of the terms used to describe interactions between the different professions within a learning context.

Context

As early as 1998, the World Health Organization (WHO) highlighted that if health professionals learned together, and learned to collaborate as students, they would be more likely to work together effectively in clinical or work-based teams. The international trend continues. In 2010, a widely researched and consulted framework was produced by the World Health Organization fully endorsing interprofessional education to support collaborative clinical practice (World Health Organization, 2010). The framework suggests that

Figure 1. Definitions used to describe the interaction between the different professions

Interprofessional education is defined by the Centre for Advancement of Interprofessional Education (2006) as occurring 'when two or more professions learn with, from and about each other to improve collaboration and the quality of care … and includes all such learning in academic and work-based settings before and after qualification, adopting an inclusive view of "professional".'

Interprofessional learning is a term often used interchangeably with interprofessional education. Both involved active engagement of learners from different professions learning together. The learning is based on an exchange of knowledge, understanding, attitudes or skills with an explicit aim of improving collaboration and health care outcomes (Freeth, 2007)

Multiprofessional learning, sometimes called shared learning or common learning, is where one or more students or professionals learn alongside one another. The learning may be around acquisition of a clinical skill or knowledge, learners may occupy the same physical space and use the same learning materials.

Uni-professional learning: in which students learn together as a single group, e.g. nurses, doctors, dentists, midwives, allied health professionals or social workers, and do not learn with or alongside other professional groups.

Teamworking: 'a considered action carried out by two or more individuals jointly, concurrently or sequentially. It implies common agreed goals, clear awareness of and respect for others' roles and functions.' (Boyd and Horne, 2008)

Collaboration: 'an interprofessional process of communication and decision-making that enables the separate and shared knowledge and skills of healthcare providers to synergistically influence the ways client/ patient care and broader community health services are provided' (Way et al, 2002).

safe, effective health care relies on developing a collaborative, practice-ready workforce.

There is overwhelming evidence that a failure of health and social care professionals to work together and communicate with each other can have tragic consequences for individuals (Laming Report, 2003; Quinney, 2006). Despite the lack of robust 'evidence' that interprofessional learning contributes to more effective collaborative practice and improved patient and client outcomes, there are clear policy drivers from governments to encourage collaborative practice and partnership working.

Drivers for interprofessional learning

The main driver behind the development and implementation of interprofessional learning is to help improve health and social care services. This was in the wake of shifting service delivery patterns (including more care in the community, shorter inpatient stays and changes in professional roles) and a response to some high profile cases in which vulnerable people (often children and young people) 'fell through the net' (Colwell Report, 1974; Laming Report, 2003).

Interprofessional learning helps to promote a more positive attitude between healthcare professionals, to assist with the successful implementation of new policies and guidelines across disciplines and departments, and to improve communication and the environment in which healthcare professionals operate. Faresjo (2006) also suggests that economic drivers also support collaboration and partnership working, particularly in areas where healthcare resources are scarce, commenting that 'in such cases, it is essential that health and social professionals work together in order to supply sufficient care within available resources'.

Principles of interprofessional education

The Centre for the Advancement of Interprofessional Education identified seven principles 'to guide the provision and commissioning of IPE [interprofessional education] and to assist in its development and evaluation'.

The principles 'draw on the IPE [interprofessional education] literature, evidence base and the experience of CAIPE members, underpinned by values common to all health care professionals including a commitment to equal opportunities and positive regard for difference, diversity and individuality' (Centre for the Advancement of Interprofessional Education, 2006).

The Centre for the Advancement of Interprofessional Education's vision is that when interprofessional education works well, it:

1. Improves the quality of care
2. Focuses on the needs of service users and carers
3. Involves service users and carers
4. Encourages professions to learn, with, from and about each other
5. Respects the integrity and contribution of each profession
6. Enhances practice within professions
7. Increases professional satisfaction.

Interprofessional learning might help counter some of the potential for resentment that shared (or multiprofessional) learning might engender in its participants by active engagement of different groups with one another. However, multiprofessional learning should not be seen be seen as a subset of or step towards interprofessional education, particularly when the learning involves students from diverse professional groups. Both types of learning can exist alongside one another, many of which are at pre-registration levels, particularly in the early or foundation years where much of the basic science or communications skills learning might be shared learning. Sometimes this is with the specific aim of encouraging students to work together and learn about one another's practice, but often it is to provide students with a common foundation or baseline level of learning so as to provide them with a range of options at the next stage of learning.

Communities of practice and interprofessional learning

A concept which links closely with interprofessional learning in its collaborative approach is that of the community of practice. Simply, a community of practice can be described as a group of people who work together to achieve a common goal. The process of working together and sharing knowledge and resources can lead to an enriched learning experience as people are exposed to new ways of thinking and problem solving.

In the clinical workplace, a community of practice could be a healthcare team assigned to a particular patient. That team has been charged with the task of providing an appropriate healthcare management plan and could include in its membership specialists, consultants, surgeons, nurses, medical students, nursing students, healthcare assistants and administrative staff. Each member brings to the community of practice his/her own set of skills and knowledge and through consultation, discussion and general interaction with one another provides a substantial body of knowledge and skills which they can all draw upon. Interprofessional learning can help a community of practice to work more effectively and to prepare its members for participation in interprofessional teams.

Learning theory

The rationale for interprofessional learning is not only underpinned by service demands around teamworking, shared knowledge, professional development and collaboration, but also by learning theories. Skillfully facilitated and planned interprofessional learning can use 'constructive friction', creative conflict and the learning 'edge' to promote change, stimulate debate and discussion, and promote professional and personal development (Freeth, 2007).

Positive experiences of working and learning in mixed groups validates this hypothesis but, as Carpenter and Hewstone (1996) remind us, this is not always so easy to manage in practice. Media and other professional stereotypes, difficulties in timetabling (particularly in clinical or other work-based placements), apportioning costs, finding appropriately skilled (and credible) facilitators, finding common, meaningful assessments and ensuring the professionals graduate against their own professional standards may all conspire against the wide implementation of interprofessional learning activities.

Interprofessional learning and clinical teaching

Interprofessional learning needs to be embedded in the curriculum rather than seen as an 'add on' as it would be easy to cut when budgets are tight. It is not always simple, however, to champion interprofessional learning across different professions, departments and organizations. Some practical ideas that teachers might introduce into day-to-day teaching to promote and raise awareness of interprofessional learning include the following:

- Introduction of a new clinical protocol, approach or technique
- Case conferences (these are often multi-disciplinary, but more emphasis could be placed on learning from other professionals)
- Bringing learners from different professions together in structured formal sessions around specific topics or inviting learners from other professions to sessions which traditionally have been for single professions. Teaching modes might include lectures, seminars, tutorials, case studies and scenarios or problem-based learning
- Involving learners from different professions to work together in clinical situations (such as the clinic, consulting room, theatre, ward, community, home visits) to learn together and share experiences and perspectives on patient care or understanding of situations

- Promoting informal interprofessional learning, while providing opportunities for discussion, sharing of knowledge and learning from other professions.

Clinical skills acquisition lends itself well to interprofessional working, particularly in the latter years of the undergraduate course or in postgraduate contexts, such as anaesthetics, operating theatres, clinics or day centres. Guided by the principle 'learning from one another', rather than 'with one another', learning can use a range of interprofessional clinical scenarios. Such scenarios can be led by an interprofessional team, coordinated by an interprofessional skills teacher. In focusing on learning as a team to address patient care, participants can develop mutual respect and appreciation of the difficulties each may face when dealing with the acutely sick patient.

The role of the teacher

The teacher is instrumental in ensuring that interprofessional learning is effective at many levels: at the level of the curriculum (design and balance of activities), timetabling, allocation of resources, consideration of power relationships between different professional and academic groups and selection of appropriate activities for interprofessional learning. Once higher level decisions have been made to implement interprofessional learning activities, the teacher is also responsible for what goes on in the learning environment itself.

Lindqvist and Reeves' (2007) research on the facilitator's role provides some insight into the role of facilitating interprofessional learning and explores some of the elements that lead to successful facilitation of interprofessional learning. Results suggest that facilitators feel that in order to be effective, they need to be able to 'display a range of attributes including enthusiasm, humour and empathy'.

Some suggested guidelines for classroom management of interprofessional groups include:

- Encourage learning from rather than learning with one another
- Make sure you have an adequate, diverse and equal mix of professionals
- Ensure the majority of a session has relevance to all participants
- Use the skills, knowledge and expertise of all the participants through carefully selected activities
- Do not let one group dominate discussion and ideas
- Challenge stereotyping and negative views.

Assessment

Consideration of assessment of interprofessional learning raises a number of questions.

First, should interprofessional learning be assessed at all? Is it assessable? And if it should or can, then:

- How can interprofessional learning be assessed equitably, reliably and with validity?
- How can we develop assessments that work across different courses and professional groups and that tie in with different learning outcomes and assessment patterns?
- What should be in these assessments, what form should they take and where in the curricula should they be situated?
- Who assesses interprofessional learning? Should these be discipline-based teachers or do we need specialist interprofessional learning teachers?

With all these questions, it is unsurprising that, although there are many interprofessional learning initiatives in terms of learning activities, there has been little written about assessment as it presents one of the more difficult challenges to implementing successful interprofessional learning in the clinical setting.

Freeth (2007) suggests that the key concept underpinning assessment of interprofessional learning is that of 'constructive alignment' (Biggs and Tang, 2007), in which all aspects of the curriculum: learning outcomes, educational or learning objectives, course design, teaching and learning activities, assessment and evaluation, are aligned so that there is a clear relationship between all aspects. Morison and Stewart (2005) point out the need to develop and use agreed interprofessional learning standards or learning outcomes as the basis for developing relevant assessments. So, the consequence of this is that if we teach interprofessional learning, we should teach according to agreed learning outcomes and we should also assess it overtly. It has been suggested that for many learners, assessment drives learning and what is assessed in the formal curriculum is therefore more highly valued.

Challenges and constraints

The wide range of literature available on interprofessional learning suggests that the potential benefits are great, not only to patients or clients, but also to learners, educators and other stakeholders. It seems that the workplace, including the clinical environment, would be an appropriate place to bring learners together in interprofessional groups or teams. After all, they are working together collaboratively and so learning together would seem logical. However, implementing interprofessional learning poses many challenges to teachers, clinicians and practitioners and to educational managers and planners. Headrick et al (1998) list a number of barriers to interprofessional collaboration and education:

- Differences in history and culture
- Historical intraprofessional and interprofessional rivalries
- Differences in language and jargon
- Differences in schedules and professional routines
- Varying levels of preparation, qualifications and status
- Differences in requirements, regulations and norms of professional education
- Fears of diluted professional identity
- Differences in accountability, payment and rewards
- Concerns regarding clinical responsibility.

In clinical and professional learning contexts, Soklaridis et al (2007) note the importance for future doctors to learn from non-doctor role models and teachers and that interprofessional learning may well involve challenging differential power relations and differences (the 'us and them') between health professions. Carpenter and Hewstone (1996) evaluated a course for student doctors and social workers based on shared learning. They highlighted the potential for power differentials with a number of participants feeling that their learning was compromised, but for different reasons. Mandy et al (2004) examined whether interprofessional education had any effect on professional stereotypes held by first year undergraduate physiotherapy and podiatry students. One of their findings was that early implementation of interprofessional learning appears to reinforce stereotypes, this might be based on deep-rooted psychology. If so, undoing the stereotypes that exist within professional groups is more complicated than previously thought.

Conclusions

This chapter has introduced some of the key principles and ideas around interprofessional learning in the light of an emerging body of literature. Some of the challenges for clinical teachers are also considered. Interprofessional learning is an area of teaching and learning which many teachers feel intuitively that 'should work' but it needs careful planning. If teachers are going to implement interprofessional learning in their everyday practice then it is helpful to keep in mind that effective interprofessional learning is good educational practice 'with a twist', the twist being the active involvement of two or more groups of professionals in learning from, with and about one another.

KEY POINTS

- Interprofessional learning involves learners from two or more professional groups learning from, with and about one another.

- Interprofessional learning needs to be championed by individual teachers and built into curriculum design and strategy.

- Many opportunities for implementing interprofessional learning exist in the workplace, both formal and informal.

- Planning and preparation is essential and interprofessional learning sessions need to be relevant to all learners.

- Challenges for implementing interprofessional learning include timetabling and logistics, confronting professional stereotypes and different regulatory demands.

References

Biggs J, Tang C (2007) *Teaching for Quality Learning at University*. 3rd edn. Open University Press, Maidenhead

Boyd M, Horne W (2008) Primary Health Care in New Zealand: Teamworking and collaborative practice – Interprofessional learning 2008, Auckland, April/May 2008. Waitemata District Health Board, Auckland

Carpenter J, Hewstone M (1996) Shared learning for doctors and social workers: evaluation of a programme. *British Journal of Social Work* **26**: 239–57

Centre for the Advancement of Interprofessional Education (2006) Defining interprofessional education. www.caipe.org.uk/about-us/defining-ipe/ (accessed 13 July 2010)

Colwell Report (1974) *Report of the committee of enquiry into the care and supervision provided in relation to Maria Colwell*. HMSO, London

Faresjo T (2006) Interprofessional education – to break boundaries and build bridges. *Rural and Remote Health* **6**: 602

Freeth D (2007) *Interprofessional learning*. Understanding Medical Education series. ASME, Edinburgh:

Headrick LA, Wilcock PM, Batalden PB (1998) Interprofessional working and continuing medical education. *BMJ* **316**(7133): 771–4

Laming Report (2003) *The Victoria Climbié Inquiry: Report of an inquiry by Lord Laming*. HMSO, London (www.victoria-climbie-inquiry.org.uk accessed 10 June 2008)

Lindqvist SM, Reeves S (2007) Facilitators' perceptions of delivering interprofessional education: a qualitative study. *Med Teach* **29**(4): 403–5

Mandy A, Milton C, Mandy P (2004) Professional stereotyping and interprofessional education. *Learning in Health and Social Care* **3**(3): 154–70

Morison SL, Stewart MC (2005) Developing interprofessional assessment. *Learning in Health and Social Care* **4**(4): 192–202

Quinney A (2006) *Collaborative Social Work Practice*. Learning Matters, Exeter

Soklaridis S, Oandasan I, Kimpton S (2007) Family health teams: can health professionals learn to work together? *Can Fam Physician* **53:** 1198–9

Way DO, Busing N, Jones L (2002) *Implementing Strategies: collaboration in primary care – family doctors and nurse practitioners delivering shared care*. Ontario College of Family Physicians, Toronto

World Health Organization (1998) *Learning together to work together for health*. WHO, Geneva

World Health Organization (2010) *Framework for action on interprofessional education and collaborative practice*. Health Professions Network Nursing and Midwifery Office within the Department of Human Resources for Health. WHO, Geneva

e-learning for clinical teachers

Iain Doherty and Judy McKimm

Clinical teachers teach diverse groups of learners who are increasingly familiar with learning through an online environment. e-learning provides huge opportunities for enhancing clinical teaching and facilitating communication. However, to be effective, e-learning must be grounded within sound educational approaches.

This chapter explores the role of and potential for introducing a range of technologies in clinical teaching, set within the context of a framework of principles for good teaching practice. It looks at how teachers might select and implement technologies appropriately when planning teaching sessions, writing learning objectives and designing learning activities and assessments.

What is e-learning?

e-learning is now very much part of mainstream health professions' education. Students and trainees are very familiar with using computers and other technologies as part of their day-to-day life, in healthcare management and in education. In this chapter e-learning refers to electronically-mediated learning in a digital format (using computers and the internet) to enhance or facilitate teaching and learning (Bullen, 2006). This definition covers the use of technologies to supplement face-to-face teaching through to distance teaching opportunities in which teacher and student may never meet face-to-face such as *British Medical Journal Learning* (Walsh and Dillner, 2003).

Ellaway and Masters (2008) distinguish between e-learning, e-teaching and e-assessment, highlighting that e-learning is not just about the content and the delivery of teaching, but is a pedagogical approach that aims 'to be flexible, engaging and learner-centred: one that encourages interaction (staff:staff, staff:student, student:student) collaboration and communication'.

Although there are huge opportunities to enhance clinical teaching through e-learning a number of challenges exist in addition to determining pedagogical aspects. Teachers will need to be familiar with the range of innovations available so that they can select appropriate means of developing content, facilitating the process of learning and enabling communication. Other challenges include becoming familiar with new systems, processes and online environments, making time to filter through and select appropriate materials, having time to support learners as they use e-learning and keeping materials and activities up to date.

The educational context

'The challenge for medical educators is to be aware of the new changes and to consider how the latest technology can be used to enhance learning' (Sandars and Haythornthwaite, 2007).

Technological innovations appear tempting, particularly when students are learning at a distance and when there is such an array of possibilities available. However, if we are going to talk about e-learning in an educationally useful way we need to start by talking first about teaching and learning. Taking an approach that first identifies and looks for answers to educational challenges will be more likely to result in the appropriate use of technologies (Laurillard, 2008). Technology must take second place to good practice in education, hovering 'shyly in the wings, ready to lend its power, but only as needed' (Ahmed, 2003).

Three models or frameworks help us think about the place of e-learning in clinical teaching:
- The 'seven principles' of good teaching practice
- Distinguishing between the 'content' and the 'process' of e-learning
- 'Constructive alignment'.

The 'seven principles'

Chickering and Gamson (1987) introduced the seven principles for good practice in undergraduate education, according to which, good educational practice:
1. Encourages contact between students and faculty
2. Develops reciprocity and cooperation among students
3. Encourages active learning
4. Gives prompt feedback
5. Emphasizes time on task

6. Communicates high expectations
7. Respects diverse talents and ways of learning.

Although devised for undergraduate education, these principles are relevant to all learning situations. We can easily see how the principles could be achieved in face-to-face teaching, where teacher and learners are physically located in the same space (such as a classroom) at the same time. For example, a session might begin with the teacher communicating his/her high expectations by outlining learning objectives and defining the standards to be met in order to pass an assignment. At the same time the teacher might clarify time on task in relation to completion of learning activities and due dates for assignments.

Contact between teachers and learners can be encouraged by the teacher setting aside additional time during which he/she is available to talk to learners. Active learning can be encouraged by group-based learning activities based on collaborative research, which also encourages reciprocity and cooperation between learners. Requiring individual learners to take a lead in specific activities and building on learners' needs is one way in which the teacher can demonstrate respect for diverse talents and ways of learning. Prompt and timely feedback on progress or areas for development can be given while activities are being carried out or in one-to-one tutorials.

There is no point in introducing a technology just because it is available or for the sake of innovating. 'The novelty factor can often cause us to be tempted to implement the latest and greatest technology, sometimes without thinking carefully enough about whether or not this is actually going to result in meaningful learning' (Lee, 2005). A straightforward way to judge the potential value of a technology is to consider the seven principles and to ask how the technologies might help in adding value, realizing the principles in practice and achieving educational outcomes that would not otherwise have been possible (Gamson, 1995; Chickering and Ehrmann, 1996).

Many clinical teachers are running a busy service and may teach diverse groups of students and trainees. Putting the principles into practice may be more difficult in clinical settings than in a university setting where teaching sessions for groups of learners are clearly timetabled. Here, e-learning might help to 'scaffold' the learning, through providing a common set of learning materials, links to library resources or by enabling group discussion or collaboration to occur without the need for teacher and learners to be in the same room, or even working at the same time. One advantage of e-learning is that learners and teachers can work independently and communicate asynchronously (not in real time) through discussion boards or email. Or teachers and/or learners may communicate in real time (from their own homes or other workplaces) through chat rooms, instant messaging or Skype. Such 'classrooms without walls' can provide useful learning spaces for trainees and students who might find it difficult to meet in real time.

Content and process

Another way of thinking about how to incorporate e-learning is to distinguish between whether you are aiming to support learners through providing access to content using e-learning (e.g. course materials, links to other websites, online databases) and/or whether you aim to use e-learning to support the learning process. Of course, many programmes aim to do both, but the expectations and choice of technologies used and the types of activities selected will be shaped by your overall aim as a teacher and your students' learning needs.

e-learning content includes curriculum content, course materials, e-journals, e-books and other resources available through an e-library or online database, commercial materials, the internet (e.g. via Google, Google Scholar or Wikipedia), reusable learning objects, audio and video materials (such as clinical recordings) or podcasts or RSS (really simple syndication) feeds (Ellaway and Masters, 2008; Morris and McKimm, 2009). Learners expect tangible benefits from using information and communication technology and expect unrestricted access to resources, information and networks, however, they also expect face-to-face interaction to form a large part of their educational experience (Joint Information Systems Committee, 2008). For clinical learners who need to work and learn from patients, this is vital.

Contact between clinical teachers and learners (and the learners themselves) can be limited by teacher availability and pressures on students' or trainees' time (Issenberg and Scalese, 2007). Earlier versions of the World Wide Web – now referred to as Web 1.0 (Boulos and Wheeler, 2007) – were repositories for information, enabling access to information from anywhere and at any time, and facilitated communication through email and other means. The use of Web 1.0 technologies such as email, a chat room or a discussion board can increase opportunities for contact and supplement face-to-face contact. The less face-to-face contact time there is between teacher and learner (e.g. in distance learning programmes where technologies provide the only means of contact) the more crucial it is that technologies are used appropriately to facilitate contact and communication.

Web 2.0, although difficult to define (Anderson, 2007), is seen as a World Wide Web characterized by new applications and services which have created what is known as an architecture of participation and collaboration (Doherty, 2008). Users of the web can now create and co-create content,

Table 13.1. Web 2.0 services and applications

Categorization	Explanation	Application or service
Blog	An online personal journal or web log	http://www.blogger.com
Wiki	A collaboratively authored website	http://www.wikispaces.com
Social Bookmarking	A system for storing bookmarks on a remote server and to share bookmarks with other users of the system	http://delicious.com
Multimedia Sharing	Services that facilitate the storage and sharing of multimedia content	http://www.youtube.com
Social Networking	Professional and social network ing sites thatfacilitate meeting people, finding like minds, sharing	http://www.ning.com

share content and collaborate much more easily through tools such as blogs, wikis, social bookmarking services, multimedia sharing services and social networking spaces (Anderson, 2007) *(Table 13.1)*.

Although many e-learning activities directly replicate face-to-face activities (group discussions, reading articles), other activities can be significantly enhanced through e-learning which can facilitate collaboration and cooperation between learners. For example, using the web to deliver a clinical case scenario, supported by online resources (such as simulations, test results, scans and images), would make the case available at any time and place for a group of learners as long as they had internet access. Using Web 2.0 tools such as a wiki environment would allow each learner to discuss the case without having to physically meet with others. This flexibility is important for learners who find face-to-face meetings difficult because, for example, of the demands of a part time job or shiftwork.

We might assume that learners who have grown up in the digital age would be driving e-learning. However, 'not all learners are confident users of the wide range of learning technologies available, and there is an increasing literature that highlights the challenges for learners (many of which are similar to those identified by clinical teachers)' (Morris and McKimm, 2009).

Constructive alignment

So far we have looked specifically at principles for good practice for individual teachers but we also need to ensure that technologies are successfully integrated at a course level in terms of a coherent teaching plan. A curriculum, course or 'lesson' should have an aim, specific learning objectives or outcomes, learning activities designed to enable students to realize the learning objectives, valid and reliable assessments designed to measure student learning (Atherton, 2005) (see Chapter 3) and evaluation to measure the effect of the intervention. These are the basic elements of 'the educational paradigm' (*see Figure 11.2 on page 105*) which, guided and informed by educational principles (Matheson, 2009), should be linked together so as to enable 'constructive alignment' (Biggs, 1996).

Planning and implementing e-learning activities

A consideration of these elements helps us see how technologies might be appropriately integrated into teaching at a course and/or curriculum level (Elgort et al, 2008). *Figure 13.2* provides an illustrative example using a template developed to support the creation of flexible and distance teaching materials to ensure constructive alignment. This example is informed by the teaching and learning seven principles, defines teaching and learning methods and indicates how e-learning content and process might be introduced.

In this example, the teacher uses e-learning to facilitate the group learning process, providing supporting content and links as well as structuring the learning process to achieve the learning outcomes which are then assessed. Evaluation is important, particularly after introducing a teaching or learning innovation, in order to gauge whether learning improves as a result of the innovation and whether changes might need to be made. Evaluation of Web 2.0 tools as teaching innovations is not something that is currently happening (Elgort et al, 2008), referred to by Booth (2007) as an 'educational bypass'.

Conclusions

e-learning provides huge opportunities and potential benefits for both learners and clinical teachers, enabling access to a vast amount of resources and facilitating communication when face-to-face learning is difficult. However, it is vital to maintain the main focus on improving teaching and learning while acknowledging that new technologies can enhance and facilitate teaching and learning.

Figure 13.2. Development template for e-learning – an example.

Aims:	Learners will work collaboratively in small groups for 1 week to produce a group presentation and written individual assignment summarising the key principles of transmission, disease process and management of influenza(s) from both individual patient and public health perspectives		
Learning objectives/ outcomes:	Learners will be able to demonstrate understanding of the key principles of outcomes transmission, disease process and clinical and public health management of influenza(s)		
Methods	**Assessment**		**Evaluation**
Process: Learner role/activity, e.g. students will work collaboratively in small groups to produce a summary of the key principles of transmission, disease process and clinical and public health management of influenza(s) Process: Tutor support role, e.g. written instructions, marking schemes, course announcements, frequently asked questions page, moderation of online discussions	Formative assessment, e.g. learners present their group's summaries (online or face-to-face) Summative assessment, . e.g. written individual assignment Assignments marked in accordance with defined criteria and marking scheme, constructive feedback provided		Student feedback questionnaire on whether the content provided was helpful and/ or appropriate, any difficulties with accessing materials or links, did they feel equipped and confident in using Web 2.0 tools, how group communication worked, whether tutor support was sufficient, whether they felt that e-learning helped them to achieve the learning outcomes
Content: Resources, e.g. hard copy reference materials scanned and uploaded onto a virtual learning environment, multimedia resources such as video, audio and images, selected online links such as relevant websites, links to e-library			
Process and content: Mode of delivery, e.g. web-based learning materials, CD-based delivery of multimedia resources, online group work through a wiki, chat room or discussion board			
From Learning Technology Unit, Faculty of Medical and Health Sciences, University of Auckland			

KEY POINTS

- e-learning is now part of mainstream education for all health professions.

- The primary reasons for introducing e-learning must be concerned with meeting learners' needs and facilitating the educational process, not simply seizing on technological innovations.

- We must not assume that learners are familiar with e-learning tools, but provide support for access and use.

- Opportunities for enhancing learning through e-learning include access to a wide range of resources and information and facilitating communication.

- Challenges for teachers include working with new systems and processes as well as finding time for developing and maintaining e-learning resources.

References

Ahmed A (2003) Faculty adoption of technology: Training comes first. *Educational Technology* **March/April:** 51–3

Anderson P (2007) What is web 2.0? Ideas, technologies and implications for education. Joint Information Systems Committee. www.jisc.ac.uk/media/documents/techwatch/tsw0701b.pdf (accessed 15 May 2009)

Atherton JS (2005) Teaching and learning: *Assessment*. www.learningandteaching.info/teaching/assessment.htm (accessed 15 May 2009)

Biggs J (1996) Enhancing teaching through constructive alignment. *Higher Education* **32**: 347–64

Booth A (2007) Blogs, wikis and podcasts: The 'evaluation bypass' in action? *Health Info Libr J* **24**: 298–302

Boulos MNK, Wheeler S (2007) The emerging web 2.0 social software: An enabling suite of sociable technologies in health and health care education. *Health Info Libr J* **24**(1): 2–23

Bullen M (2006) When worlds collide: Project management and the collegial culture. In: Pasian BL, Woodill G, eds. *Plan to learn: Case studies in elearning project management*. Canadian eLearning Enterprise Alliance, Dartmouth, Nova Scotia: 169–76

Chickering AW, Ehrmann SC (1996) Implementing the seven principles: Technology as lever. *American Association for Higher Education Bulletin* **49**(2): 3–6

Chickering AW, Gamson ZF (1987) Seven principles of good practice in undergraduate education. *American Association for Higher Education Bulletin* **39**(7): 3–7

Doherty I (2008) Web 2.0: A movement within the health community. *Health Care and Informatics Review Online* **June** www.hinz.org.nz/uploads/file/Journal%20Jun08/Doherty%20P49.pdf (accessed 23 December 2009)

Elgort I, Smith AG, Toland J (2008) Is wiki an effective platform for group course work? *Australasian Journal of Educational Technology* **24**(2): 195–210

Ellaway R, Masters K (2008) AMEE Guide 32: e-learning in medical education. Part 1: Learning, teaching and assessment. *Med Teach* **30**: 455–73

Gamson ZF (1995) The seven principles for good practice in undergraduate education: A historical perspective. In: Hatfield S, ed. *The seven principles in action: Improving undergraduate education*. Anker Press, Boltn, Mass

Issenberg SB, Scalese RJ (2007) Best evidence in high-fidelity simulation: what clinical teachers need to know. *The Clinical Teacher* **4**: 73–7

Joint Information Systems Committee (2008) *Great expectations of ICT: how Higher Education institutions are measuring up: Research study conducted for the Joint Information Systems Committee* (JISC). IPSOS MORI, London

Laurillard D (2008) The teacher as action researcher: Using technology to capture pedagogic form. *Studies in Higher Education* **33**(2): 139–54

Lee M (2005) New tools for online collaboration: Blogs, wikis, rss and podcasting. *Training and Development in Australia* **32**(5): 17–20

London Deanery (2008) The educational paradigm. www.faculty.londondeanery.ac.uk/e-learning/setting-learning-objectives/the-educational-paradigm (accessed 15 May 2009)

Matheson D (2009) Learning objectives. www.nottingham.ac.uk/medical-school/tips/aims_objectives.html (accessed 15 May 2009)

Morris C, McKimm J (2009) Becoming a digital tourist: a guide for clinical teachers. *The Clinical Teacher* **6**: 51–5

Sandars J, Haythornthwaite C (2007) New horizons for e-learning in medical education: ecological and Web 2.0 perspectives. *Med Teach* **29**(4): 307–10

Walsh K, Dillner L (2003) Launching BMJ Learning. *BMJ* **327**: 1064

CHAPTER 14

Using simulation in clinical education

Kirsty Forrest and Judy McKimm

Patient simulation in all its forms is widely used in clinical education with the key aims of improving learners' competence and confidence, improving patient safety and reducing errors. Understanding its benefits, range of uses and limitations will help clinical teachers improve the learning experience.

This chapter discusses how simulation can be used in medical and health professions' education to develop and improve practical and team resource management skills and introduces the most common uses of simulation in clinical education settings.

Introduction

Simulations are a dress rehearsal of a real event where as many mistakes as possible can be made and lessons can be learned, but no one comes to harm.

People from many occupations (including athletes, actors and pilots) use simulation as part of their training. In these professions, in common with medicine, people have to perform skills in high pressure situations. The first recorded use of a medical simulator is that of a manikin created in the 17th century by a Dr Gregoire of Paris (Buck, 1991). He used a pelvis with skin stretched across it to simulate an abdomen, and with the help of a dead fetus explained assisted and complicated deliveries to midwives.

In spite of this early start, medical simulators did not gain widespread use in the following centuries, principally for reasons of cost, reluctance to adopting new teaching methods, and scepticism that what was learned from a simulator could be transferred to the actual practice. All of these reasons are still relevant today, but the combination of increased awareness of patient safety, improved technology and increased pressures on educators have promoted simulation as one option to address problems with traditional clinical skills teaching. Simulation has moved from the province of a few enthusiasts to a mainstream learning modality.

The American anaesthetist Gaba said:

'No industry in which human lives depend on the skilled performance of responsible operators has waited for unequivocal proof of the benefit of simulation before embracing it.' (Gaba, 1992)

Most junior clinicians will now be trained and assessed in simulators and the use of clinical skills or simulation laboratories is seen as routine in medical and health professions' education. Advances in technology mean that there are very lifelike simulators for patients, surgery procedures and full-scale mock-ups of wards, theatre and emergency departments. Many include software so that the simulator's reactions depend on learners' actions. There are many advantages to simulator training. The most obvious is that trainees can practice as often as they like and whenever they want (within reason) without harming a patient.

Why simulation now?

The 2008 annual report of the Chief Medical Officer, *Safer Medical Practice* (Donaldson, 2009), spelled out the importance of simulator training to improve patient safety and clinicians' performance and to enable experience to be gained without practice on patients. Four key drivers for the widespread introduction of simulation are:

1. Public expectation. The public not only expect professionals to engage in appropriate skills and simulator training, they often believe that the profession already does. Patient groups are shocked to learn that doctors frequently perform a skill for the first time on a real patient.

2. Changes in working practice. The development of new professional roles, the growth of large and complex working environments, the widespread adoption of shift systems and the rapid pace of modern health care requires clinicians to develop high order leadership, team working and communication skills. Simulation has been at the forefront of the development (and assessment) of these skills.

3. Technological developments and opportunities. The technology available to support high fidelity and simulator training has progressed rapidly in recent years. Evidence exists that the educational value from low fidelity simulators can outweigh that of high fidelity simulators as long as they are embedded within an educationally sound training programme.

4. Reduced training time. A number of changes including the European Working Time Directive have reduced the time available for clinical training; to make the best possible use of available work-based time, trainees must have prepared effectively away from the work place.

Benefits of simulation

The use of simulation in health professions' education has benefits for learners, for development of clinical practice and skills, for patients and for health systems (Riley et al, 2003). There is now a significant and growing body of evidence that simulator training is educationally effective in developing technical skills (Ziv et al 2003). As well as facilitating the acquisition of routine skills, simulation also allows safe (for the learner and the patient) exposure to rare diseases, critical incidents, near misses and crisis situations that learners may not be exposed to during clinical training. Reflecting the experience of the airline, nuclear and other high risk industries, evidence is slowly accumulating in medicine that patient safety standards and non-technical skills improve following simulator training (Beyea, 2004; McGaghie et al, 2010).

How is simulation used?

Simulation training extends from part task trainers, or procedural training to the experience of full clinical situations. *Table 14.1* lists the range of low to high fidelity simulated experiences.

For example simulated parts of the body can be used for cannulation, catheterization and rectal examination. Some skills are practiced in a wet lab where animal and human tissue can be used, for example for suturing. Basic (low fidelity) manikins are used for teaching basic and advanced life support. High fidelity manikin simulators with a vast number of programmed interactions and physiological responses can be used for individual or team scenario training.

High fidelity simulators also include those that are used for laparoscopic and endoscopic skills where virtual reality is used. Some of these sophisticated

Table 14.1. The range of simulated experiences
Games, classroom scenarios
Wet labs using human or animal tissue
Simulated patients, either actors or volunteers
Computer-generated virtual reality simulators
Manikins and models of varying complexity, from part task trainers, such as cannulation arms to 'complete' bodies such as Simman
Mock hospital facilities including a simulated operating theatre, emergency departments and wards

simulators have 'forced feedback' (haptic) systems which enable the learner to 'feel' the endoscope going around the splenic flexure.

Despite the ready availability of simulated body parts and 'kit', the integration of technical and non-technical skills is paramount in developing professional practice. In addition, to ensure patient safety, non-technical skills are an aspect of training that should be emphasized. Analyses of adverse incidents indicates that the majority of causes of errors are in the non-technical skill domain, including communication failure, team failure, poor leadership or poor decision making (Gawande et al, 2003; Mallory et al, 2003). The Scottish Clinical Simulation Centre has looked at the integration of human factors into the medical curriculum and how to access the acquisition of those skills. They have developed behavioural markers for these skills in both the anaesthetic and surgical arenas.

Kneebone et al's (2003) research programme on the integration of technical and non-technical skills includes simulation training for rectal endoscopy which uses an endoscopy simulator with a simulated patient next to the simulator. A sheet covers the patient and the trainee has to perform the task while talking and explaining to the 'patient' what he or she is doing.

Scenario simulation provides an excellent opportunity for interprofessional education with the ability to train real teams from work environments. In addition, predetermined healthcare groups deliver many of the skills required by patients during their care, but in the future who delivers these skills may well change. It is envisaged that simulation teaching will provide packages that any group could access and interact with other groups for relevant multidisciplinary situations.

Simulation and learning

The development and adoption of simulation training reflects development in theories of learning from more individually oriented activities to those that view learning as a social and cultural event. Simulations that focus on improving team performance are therefore becoming increasingly commonplace in high risk environments such as anaesthesia, surgery and emergency medicine (Gaba, 2006; Ker and Bradley, 2007; Nestel et al, 2008).

As simulation becomes an accepted part of everyday education and training for health professionals, attention is being paid to how simulation can best be used to develop technical and non-technical skills. Simulation appears to work most effectively when it is designed to meet curricular outcomes, includes realistic and relevant content, interesting and engaging learning methods and prepares learners for working in the clinical context in terms of activities, skills and competencies (Issenberg et al, 2005). *Table 14.2* lists the best practice features of simulation as identified in two systematic literature reviews.

Simulation helps skills acquisition, maintenance and assessment in the move from 'novice to expert' (Dreyfus and Dreyfus, 1985). The key element is building simulation activities into learners' progression (*Figures 14.1* and *14.2*). For example medical students must practice and master the skills and pass an assessment before embarking on clinical rotations or trainees might have to provide evidence of competence in a simulator before interacting with patients. Learners can therefore have their first encounter with patients at a higher level of technical and clinical proficiency which protects patients (Ziv et al, 2003).

Table 14.2. Best practice features of simulation
Formative feedback during simulation
An opportunity for deliberate and repetitive practice
Curriculum integration
Outcome measurement
Simulation fidelity
Skills acquisition and maintenance
Mastery learning
Transfer to practice
Team training
High stakes testing
Instructor training
Educational and professional context
A variety of conditions and range of difficulties
From Issenberg et al (2005); McGaghie et al (2010)

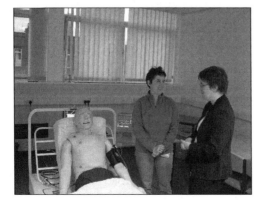

Figure 14.1. Using a simulator for learning and teaching.

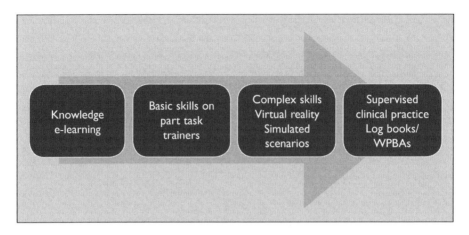

Figure 14.2. Simulation activities integrated into the learning programme.
WPBA = workplace-based assessment.

Clinicians can use simulated facilities to rehearse both challenging and routine procedures to reduce error (Yule et al, 2006). The philosophy is based on deliberate practise with appropriate feedback (both during and after the training event). Because simulation focuses primarily on skills acquisition (technical or non-technical), it is essential that learning activities are planned with clear learning outcomes and that a de-briefing or follow up stage is planned (Cumin et al, 2008).

The absence of learner feedback is the greatest single factor for ineffective simulation training. A lack of feedback may lead to:

1. Learning the wrong learning objective
2. Not realizing what the desired behaviours should be by not focusing on them
3. Not transferring skills to clinical practice
4. Spending increasing time on only one aspect of training.

A novel aspect of high fidelity simulation is the ability to play back videos of the simulated activity to an individual or team. Unlike verbal feedback from an observer there is tangible evidence of what the learner did or did not do or say. In addition, insight into how the learner behaves under stress (getting angry, withdrawal, making mistakes) is a valuable and powerful learning tool.

Deliberate practice refers to time spent on a specific activity designed to improve performance in a particular aspect of practice. Deliberate practice is a better method of acquiring expertise than simple unstructured practice (Ericsson, 2004). There is a consistent association between the amount and the quality of deliberate practice and performance in domains as varied as chess, music and sport (Ericsson and Charness, 1994). Deliberate practice means that there is effort involved as well as some form of feedback, whether through self assessment, from the simulator or observation by another person.

Short-term training courses are not the same as deliberate practice and do not have the same beneficial effects on long-term performance. Research with laparoscopic equipment has shown that structured practice with feedback improves subsequent performance in the same real-life situation (Reznick and MacRae, 2006). Deliberate practice using simulation is particularly useful for new skills, rare events or emergencies.

A lack of opportunity for practice is associated with a poor educational outcome. This is often attributed to insufficient access to the simulator, as training sessions are usually time dependent, and the simulator is often a hotly-contested resource. In addition, each learner is different, and some learners inevitably need longer or more frequent sessions with the simulator to achieve the same educational results as their co-learners.

Simulation in practice

You have found a Simman (Laerdal, Orpington, Kent) manikin within your department and you think it would be a good way to teach trainees on how to deal with critical incidents. How would you start to prepare?

Be very specific about your educational goals – sometimes it is very easy to get carried away with the technology and forget what outcomes you are after. Once you have set out your aims and objectives, be very specific about your scenarios. It is helpful to write these down as flow diagrams as this is often what the computer programs for the manikins look like. Try to anticipate student replies, think outside the box as some replies or actions can be very surprising and have an appropriate reply or action from the manikin ready (*Figure 14.3*).

Figure 14.3. Simman being used in team training. Reproduced by kind permission of Laerdal.

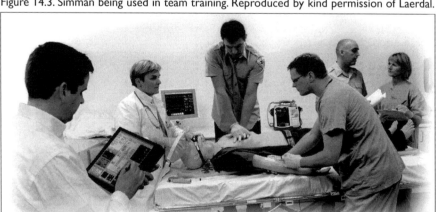

Practice running through the scenario on the manikin – this is when you find that the physical signs of the manikin that you expected sometimes are not present and you will have to adjust the scenario to maintain realism. You will be 'walking through' the scenario, gathering kit and turning the environment into a realistic set. Enrol the help of a colleague: often you need one person to run the scenario (and manikin) and the other to observe the trainee, especially when looking at non-technical skills.

Limitations of simulation

Although simulation is widespread, popular with learners and teachers and technological developments are leading to the availability of more and more complex simulators, much of the published work has been descriptive rather than grounded in evidence-based research (Issenberg et al, 2005). Contemporary research is now focussing on a more analytical, evaluative and inter-disciplinary perspective to identify how best, often costly, simulation can be used.

Simulation is not a substitute for health professionals learning with and from real patients in real clinical contexts, but is best used to teach practical or technical skills before working with patients and to replicate clinical scenarios in a safe and controlled environment (Pratt and Sachs, 2006). Gaba (2004) notes that 'simulation is a technique, not a technology'. Although the technology can become confining for some users (Kneebone and ApSimon, 2001), others remind us that we must take care that the seductive powers of the technology do not lead to a use of simulation where it leads to dependency, becomes self-referential and produces a 'new reality' (Kneebone et al, 2005; Bligh and Bleakley, 2006). Kneebone et al (2004) note that simulation must not become an end in itself, disconnected from professional practice, leading to over-confidence in learners.

Simulation must be valid. Poor validity is associated with a lack of realism. In some simulators novices can out-perform an expert, which questions the validity of that simulation. Typically this would also lead to a lack of correlation with other outcome measures.

When considering simulation activities, teachers need to think how well they can be controlled (tractability), how well they match the real world (correspondence) and how well they involve learners meaningfully (engagement). A common misconception is that high fidelity simulation is better than low fidelity. High fidelity simulation is useful for skills involving complex interactions requiring integration of cognitive and psychomotor skills coupled with interaction with others in the healthcare setting (Gaba, 2006). Maran and Glavin (2003) consider the progression from low to high fidelity simulation compared to the progression through medical education and conclude that the range of fidelity available is almost all potentially useful, but that many simulators are underused simply because of a lack of clear educational goals. Teachers therefore need to learn how to use simulation activities through faculty development and experience so as to make the most of resources and learning opportunities for their students or trainees and to integrate such activities into educational programmes, rather than being a bolt-on. Many simulation centres now offer training for teachers in the educational use of simulation.

Future directions

Policy agendas from government and professional bodies endorse, promote and fund patient simulation on a widespread scale (Donaldson, 2009). As well as helping to ensure patient safety and reduce error, simulation is also seen as an alternative means of learners acquiring clinical skills without spending time in an increasingly over-crowded clinical environment (Nursing and Midwifery Council, 2007). Educators must therefore be attentive to such agendas and ensure that simulation is complementary to learning in the clinical workplace and that learning in each context is relevant to achieving defined outcomes and developing safe, competent practitioners. It is likely that simulation will become more integrated into curricula and embedded into education and training programmes.

Opportunities for more interprofessional learning around non-technical skills and teamworking are likely to increase as more centres offer such learning opportunities although more evidence is required as to the efficacy of such training. Simulation has also been used to support new ways of working (McKimm, 2006). As health and social services change towards more integrated, patient-led approaches, we may see more use of simulation to support their introduction.

The biggest restraints to simulation training are cost and access. There are only a handful of centres across the country that can provide immersive high-fidelity simulations, the 'real' experience in mock clinical areas with all the appropriate equipment, manikins and faculty. One group has tried to address these issues by identifying the key aspects of the theatre environment that are needed for learning and then replicating these in a portable environment that can be set up in a short space of time and a small area. This ability has been coined 'distributed simulation' (Kneebone et al, 2010), where inflatable, portable theatres can be erected in places of work and simulations can be run. In addition to providing more easily accessible training, this kind of technology is much cheaper. This increasing emphasis on the ability to bring the simulation to the learner has also been replicated by other initiatives such as 'man in a van' or 'Simvan', where the equipment is mobile and taken to the learner and the simulation occurs in the van. However, both of these innovative developments still need trained faculty and a peripatetic educator to travel with the equipment.

Technological changes will also lead to much more integrated multimedia simulations such as the use of handheld devices, portable simulators and further development of virtual reality simulators.

Conclusions

Simulation is widely used to introduce and develop clinical skills and mould future behaviours in undergraduate and post-qualification education and training. There are benefits for patients and learners when simulation is used appropriately and effectively. As with any learning intervention, planning and preparation is vital; know your equipment and make sure technical support is available if required. Teachers need to ensure that simulation activities help learners to achieve defined learning outcomes, that the simulation and scenario is relevant to 'real world' learning, that feedback is built into the process and that learners are enabled to transfer the learning into the clinical context. There is no 'one size fits all' and the wide range of simulators available mean that teachers can easily incorporate some sort of simulation activity into learning. Finally, particularly for high fidelity, complex simulations, make sure that the benefits of using simulation outweigh the costs of time for faculty, technical support, space and equipment purchases.

KEY POINTS

- Simulation is widely used in health professionals' education and training.
- Simulation can help reduce error, increase patient safety and develop more competent practitioners.
- It is most effective for training in technical or practical skills and for non-technical skills in team situations.
- Simulation experiences include simple models, simulated patients, computer-based virtual reality simulators and mock clinical facilities.
- Effective simulation includes preparation, link to clear learning outcomes, deliberate practice and feedback.

References

Beyea SC (2004) Human patient simulation: a teaching strategy. *AORN Journal* **80:** 738–42

Bligh D, Bleakley A (2006) Distributing menus to hungry learners: can learning by simulation become simulation of learning? *Med Teach* **28:** 606–13

Buck GH (1991) Development of simulators in medical education. *Gesnerus* **48**(1): 7–28

Cumin D, Merry AF, Weller JM (2008) Standards for simulation. *Anaesthesia* **63:** 1281–7

Donaldson L (2009) *Annual Report of the Chief Medical Officer, 2008.* The Stationery Office, London

Dreyfus HL, Dreyfus SE (1985) *Mind over Machine: the Power of Human Intuition and Expertise in the Era of the Computer.* Free Press, New York

Ericsson KA (2004) Deliberate practice and the acquisition and maintenance of expert performance in medicine and related domains. *Acad Med* **79**(S10): S70–S81

Ericsson KA, Charness N (1994) Expert performance: its structure and acquisition. *Am Psychologist* **49:** 725–47

Gaba DM (1992) Improving anesthesiologists performance by simulating. *Anesthesiology* **76:** 491–4

Gaba DM (2004) The future vision of simulation in healthcare. *Qual Saf Health Care* **13:** i2–i10

Gaba DM (2006) *What does simulation add to teamwork training?* Agency for Healthcare Research and Quality, Rockville, Maryland (www.webmm.ahrq.gov/perspective. aspx?perspectiveID=20 accessed 7 May 2010)

Gawande AA, Zinner MJ, Studdert DM, Brennan TA (2003) Analysis of errors reported by surgeons at three teaching hospitals. *Surgery* **133:** 614–21

Issenberg SB, McGaghie WC, Petrusa E, Gordon D, Scalese RJ (2005) Features and uses of high-fidelity medical simulations that lead to effective learning: a BEME systematic review. *Med Teach* **27:** 10–28

Ker J, Bradley P (2007) *Simulation in Medical Education.* Association for the Study of Medical Education, Edinburgh

Kneebone RL, ApSimon D (2001) Surgical skills training: simulation and multimedia combined. *Med Educ* **35:** 909–15

Kneebone RL, Nestel D, Moorthy K, Taylor P, Baan S, Munz Y, Darzi A (2003) Learning the skills of flexible sigmoidoscopy – the wider perspective. *Med Educ* **37**(S1): 50–8

Kneebone RL, Scott W, Darzi A, Horrocks M (2004) Simulation and clinical practice: strengthening the relationship. *Med Educ* **38:** 1095–102

Kneebone RL, Kidd J, Nestel D et al (2005) Blurring the boundaries: scenario-based simulation in a clinical setting. *Med Educ* **39:** 580–7

Kneebone R, Arora S, King D et al (2010) Distributed simulation--accessible immersive training. *Med Educ* **32:** 65–70

Mallory S, Weller J, Bloch M, Maze M (2003) The individual, the system and medical error. *Br J Anaesth CEPD Reviews* **6***:* 179–82

Maran NJ, Glavin RJ (2003) Low- to High fidelity simulation – a continuum of medical education. *Med Educ* **37**(S1): 22–8

McGaghie WC, Issenberg SB, Petrusa ER, Scalese RJ (2010) A critical review of simulation-based medical education research: 2003–2009. *Med Educ* **44:** 50–63

McKimm J (2006) *Report to the Ways of Learning Task Group: Assignment 5 - An assessment of the benefits of simulation-based training and of learning centres for simulation based training*. Department of Health, London

Nestel DF, Black SA, Kneebone RL, Wetzel CM, Thomas P, Wolfe JHN, Darzi AW (2008) Simulated anaesthetists in high fidelity simulators for surgical training: feasibility of a training programme for actors. *Med Educ* **30:** 407–13

Nursing and Midwifery Council (2007) NMC *Circular 36/2007: Supporting direct care through simulated practice learning in the pre-registration nursing programme*. Nursing & Midwifery Council, London

Pratt SD, Sachs BP (2006) Team training: Classroom training vs high fidelity simulation? Agency for Healthcare Research and Quality, Rockville, Maryland (www.webmm.ahrq.gov/perspective.aspx?perspectiveID=20 (accessed 7 May 2010)

Reznick RK, MacRae H (2006) Teaching surgical skills - changes in the wind. *N Engl J Med* **355**(25): 2664–9

Riley RH, Grauze AM, Chinnery C, Horely RA, Trewhella NH (2003) Three years of 'CASMS': the world's busiest medical simulation centre. *Med J Aust* **179:** 626–30

Yule S, Flin R, Paterson-Brown S, Maran N (2006) Non-technical skills for surgeons in the operating room: A review of the literature. *Surgery* **139**(2): 140–9

Ziv A, Wolpe PR, Small DK, Glick S (2003) Simulation-based medical education: an ethical imperative. *Acad Med* **78:** 783–8

CHAPTER 15

Structured assessments of clinical competence

Katharine AM Boursicot

Clinical teachers are often involved in assessing clinical competence in the workplace, in universities and colleges. Assessments commonly used to formally assess clinical competence include long and short cases and the objective structured clinical examination which, if well designed, is a fair and reliable method of assessing clinical competence.

This chapter outlines the theoretical principles underlying the development of modern structured assessments of clinical competence and describes some practical aspects of designing and implementing objective structured clinical examinations (OSCEs).

Introduction

The reliable and valid assessment of clinical competence has become an increasingly important area of concern in medical education as the psychometric properties of different assessment tools have been researched and better understood.

While Miller's model of professional competence (Miller, 1990) illustrates that competence is underpinned by a thorough base of specialist medical knowledge, the term clinical competence encompasses other professional practice elements such as history taking and clinical examination skills, skills in practical procedures, doctor–patient communication, problem-solving ability and management skills, relationships with colleagues and ethical behaviour.

As written tests do not assess clinical skills, the assessment of clinical competence has historically involved the direct observation of candidates by professional colleagues. A variety of formats for assessing clinical competence has developed over the years including the 'classic' long and short case formats and newer methods such as the OSCE.

Long and short cases

In the traditional long case the holistic appraisal of the examinee's ability to interact with, assess and manage a real patient is a laudable goal and contributes to the face validity of this method. However, in recent years there has been much criticism of this approach related to variations in examiner stringency, unstructured questioning and global marking without anchor statements and patient variability – in information disclosure, demeanour, comfort and health. Perhaps more importantly, examinees' clinical skills may vary significantly across cases, so that assessing examinees on one patient cannot not provide generalizable estimates of a candidate's overall ability (Norcini, 2001, 2002).

Although apparently similar to an OSCE in providing a larger range of short cases, the differences between short cases and an OSCE are that different students rarely see the same patients, cases differ in their complexity, the same two assessors examine the student at each case, the examination is not structured and the examiners are free to ask any questions they wish. These factors result in poor reliability of this method and OSCEs have superseded this genre of assessment.

Objective structured clinical examinations

The OSCE is an assessment format in which the candidates rotate sequentially around a series of structured cases located in 'stations', at each of which specific tasks have to be performed, usually involving a clinical skill, such as history taking or examination of a patient, or a practical skill. The marking scheme for each station is structured and determined in advance. There is a different examiner and a time limit for each station. The basic structure of an OSCE may be varied in timing for each station, use of checklist or rating scale for scoring, use of clinician or standardized patient as examiner, use of real patients or manikins, but the fundamental principle is that every candidate has to complete the same assignments in the same amount of time and is marked according to a structured marking schedule.

The use of OSCEs in the quantitative assessment of competence has become widespread in the field of undergraduate and postgraduate medical education since they were originally described (Harden and Gleeson, 1979). The main reasons are the high reliability of this assessment format and the equity that results from all candidates being presented with the same test. Some characteristics of a good OSCE are listed in *Table 15.1*.

Table 15.1. What makes a good objective structured clinical examination?
Blueprinting: ensure the test content maps across the learning objectives of the course
Station development and piloting: writing stations that function well
Examiner training: engage the examiners, consistency of marking contributes to the reliability
Simulated patient training: consistent performance ensures each candidate is presented with the same challenge
Organization: make detailed plans well in advance

Reliability

Essentially the OSCE was developed to address the inherent unreliability of classical long and short cases. OSCEs are more reliable than unstructured observations in three main ways:

1. Structured marking schedules allow for more consistent scoring by examiners according to pre-determined criteria
2. Candidates have to perform a number of different tasks across clinical, practical and communication skill domains – this wider sampling across different cases and skills results in a more reliable picture of a candidate's overall competence
3. As the candidates move through all the stations, each is examined by a number of different examiners, so multiple independent observations are collated. Individual examiner bias is thus attenuated.

To enhance reliability, it is better to have more stations with one examiner per station than fewer stations with two examiners per station (van der Vleuten and Swanson, 1990).

Validity

'Content' validity is determined by how well the sampling of skills matches the learning objectives of the course or degree for which that OSCE is designed (Downing, 2003). The best way to ensure an adequate spread of sampling is to use a blueprint.

Educational impact

The impact on students' learning resulting from a testing process is sometimes referred to as 'consequential' validity. It is well recognized that students focus on their assessments rather than the learning objectives of the course. Explicit, clear learning objectives aligned with clinical skills assessment content and format can be a very effective way of encouraging students to learn the desired clinical competencies.

There is a danger in the use of detailed checklists as this may encourage students to memorize the steps in a checklist rather than learn and practice the skill. Rating scale marking schedules encourage students to learn and practice skills more holistically.

Blueprinting

Blueprinting is a powerful tool which helps to focus the OSCE designers on the exact nature of what they wish to test and to relate this to the learning outcomes *(Table 15.2)*. Once the blueprint or framework for an OSCE is agreed *(Figure 15.1)*, the individual stations can be planned and classified according to this blueprint. This ensures adequate sampling across subject area and skill, in terms of numbers of stations covering each skill and the spread over the subjects or systems of the course being tested.

Station development

It is important to write the station material well in advance of the examination date so that the stations can be reviewed and tried out before the actual assessment. Station material should include:

- Construct: a statement of what that station is supposedly testing, e.g. this station tests the candidate's ability to examine the peripheral vascular system
- Clear instructions for the candidate: to inform the candidate exactly what task he/she should perform at that station
- Clear instructions for the examiners: to help the examiner at that station to understand his/her role and conduct the station properly. Include a copy of the candidate instructions
- List of equipment required
- Personnel requirements: whether the station requires a real patient or a simulated patient and the details of such individuals (age, gender, ethnicity)
- Simulated patient scenario: if the station requires a particular role to be played
- Marking schedule: this should include the important aspects of

Table 15.2. How to construct an objective structured clinical examination blueprint

Review the curriculum learning outcomes
Decide on the domains of skills to be tested
Map the domains against the learning objectives
Sampling: decide on the proportion of stations in each section
Calculate your total testing time; ensure appropriate time is allowed for the task at each station

Figure 15.1. Example of objective structured clinical examination blueprint.

System	History	Explanation	Examination	Procedures
Cardio-vascular	Chest pain	Discharge drugs	Cardiac	Blood pressure measurement
Respiratory	Haemoptysis		Respiratory	Peak flow
Gastro-intestinal	Abdominal pain	Gastroscopy	Abdominal	Rectal examinin-nation
Reproductive	Amenorrhoea	Abnormal smear	Cervical smear	
Nervous	Headache		Eyes	Ophthalmoscopy
Musculo-skeletal	Backache		Hip	
Generic	Preoperative assessment	Consent for post-mortem		Intravenous can-nulation

the skill being tested, a scoring scheme for each item and how long the station should last. The marking schedule can be either in a checklist format or a rating scale (*Figure 15.2*). Items can be grouped into three broad categories: process skills (e.g. rapport, questioning and listening), content skills (e.g. appropriate medical or technical steps or aspects of the task or skill being tested) or management skills (appropriate set questions in specific relation to the case).

Simulated patients

It is best to use well-trained simulated patients to give consistent performances in communication skills stations. It is desirable to have people across a range of ages and ethnicities as well as a balanced gender mix. Training and monitoring simulated patients is essential to ensure consistent performance – a significant factor in the reliability of the examination.

Figure 15.2. Global ratings vs checklist scores.

When objective structured clinical examinations were first introduced, extensive detailed checklists of each step of a clinical task were produced for each station. Checklists often focused on easily measured aspects of the clinical encounter and the more subtle but critical factors in clinical performance were overlooked or ignored.

The use of rating scales to assess the performance of clinical skills has been shown to be reliable when used by expert examiners (Cohen et al, 1991). Examiner training can improve their reliability further (Hodges, 2003).

It is more effective to use checklists to assess technical skills in the earlier stages of learning (at the 'novice' end of the learning trajectory) and to use rating scales to assess more complex skills, especially with increasing levels of professional competence (Arnold, 2002; Hodges et al, 2002).

Real patients

Patients do not always give the same history repeatedly; they can become tired or unwell and may develop new signs and symptoms or even lose old clinical findings; however, they can be a most valuable resource and need to be treated as such. Using real patients in OSCEs adds greatly to the validity of the assessment. Ideally patients should be used to assess the detection of common chronic clinical signs. For each clinical sign assessed you will need several patients and even the most stoical patient should not be expected to be examined by more than 10 students in the course of a day. Ideally patients should be swapped in and out of a station to allow them to have sufficient rest time.

Examiners

OSCEs require large numbers of examiners: this can be a strength, as candidates are observed and scored by clinicians, but also one of its potential weaknesses, as inconsistency between examiners will reduce the fairness and reliability of an OSCE.

Considerable resources should be devoted to examiner training. Training sessions should cover the principles of OSCEs and the role of examiners, i.e. to assess and not to teach or conduct vivas, to adhere to marking schedules, and respect the role of the simulated patient. Training can usefully involve both the marking of pre-recorded or role-played OSCE stations, after which the marking is reviewed with the clinicians.

Practical considerations

The smooth running of OSCEs is highly dependent on the detail of the practical arrangements made in advance and it is worth putting some effort into this to ensure a satisfactory day of examinations. There are many aspects to consider and these are covered extensively by Boursicot et al (2007).

Conclusions

Assessment of clinical competence is a crucial part of the basis on which decisions are made about the ability of clinicians and doctors in training. Any method of assessing clinical skills should be considered in the context of a wider programme of assessment, which should include the assessment of knowledge, clinical examination skills, practical procedure skills, doctor–patient communication, problem-solving ability, management skills, and relationships with colleagues as well as professional attitudes and behaviour.

One of the most important aspects of assessing clinical skills is the range of sampling across a candidate's skill base; this has to be taken into account when designing any assessment. OSCEs can assess clinical, communication and practical skills but are still situated in the context of an examination setting. To assess doctors in the context of their professional practice requires the use of different formats in the work place.

The author would like to acknowledge Trudie Roberts and Bill Burdick on the Understanding Medical Education booklet, OSCEs and other assessments of clinical competence, on which a large part of this chapter is based.

KEY POINTS

- Objective structured clinical examinations (OSCEs) are widespread in the assessment of clinical competence.
- OSCEs are a fair and reliable method of assessing clinical skills.
- OSCEs should be blueprinted to learning outcomes.
- Developing high quality OSCE stations takes time and effort.
- Training of simulated patients and examiners is essential.
- Authenticity is important for test validity.

References

Arnold L (2002) Assessing professional behavior: yesterday, today, and tomorrow. *Acad Med* **77**(6): 502–15

Boursicot KAM, Roberts TE, Burdick WP (2007) *OSCEs and other Assessments of Clinical Competence*. ASME, Edinburgh

Cohen R, Rothman AI, Poldre P, Ross J (1991) Validity and generalizability of global ratings in an objective structured clinical examination. *Acad Med* **66**(9): 545–8

Downing SM (2003) Validity: on the meaningful interpretation of assessment data. *Med Educ* **37**(9): 830–7

Harden RM, Gleeson FA (1979) Assessment of clinical competence using an objective structured clinical examination (OSCE). *Med Educ* **13**(1): 41–54

Hodges B (2003) Analytic global OSCE ratings are sensitive to level of training. *Med Educ* **37**(11): 1012–16

Hodges B, McNaughton N, Regehr G, Tiberius R, Hanson M (2002) The challenge of creating new OSCE measures to capture the characteristics of expertise. *Med Educ* **36**(8): 742–8

Miller G (1990) The assessment of clinical skills/competence/performance. *Acad Med* **65**(9 suppl): S63–S67

Norcini JJ (2001) The validity of long cases. *Med Educ* **35**(8): 720–1

Norcini JJ (2002) The death of the long case? *BMJ* **324**(7334): 408–9

van der Vleuten CPM, Swanson DB (1990) Assessment of clinical skills with standardized patients: State of the Art. *Teach Learn Med* **2**(2): 58–76

CHAPTER 16

Appraisal

Doug Parkin and Judy McKimm

Appraisal is a formal process for health professionals at all levels, including those in training, which supports professional development and stimulates improvements in clinical practice. Appraisal skills are fundamental to the process of educational supervision.

This chapter focuses on the general principles of appraisal, highlighting how effective appraisal can help improve patient care and support continuing professional development as well as noting some of the specific tasks and activities relating to the appraisal of health professionals working in the NHS. It discusses appraisal skills: the importance of preparation, how to structure and manage the appraisal meeting and the key role of self-assessment as well as the outcomes of appraisal, looking at work and personal development objectives and development planning.

What is appraisal?

Appraisal is a structured process for improving future clinical, managerial and educational performance while reviewing past performance. The main beneficiary is the person being appraised. The 'job-holder' receives constructive feedback on his/her job performance in a motivational process that results in an action plan for future performance and development also known as a personal development plan. Ineffective or poor appraisals usually stem from a lack of understanding of what they are for, what they should achieve, and who should benefit and how.

As understanding of the manager's role has changed, moving away from 'command and control' and towards 'lead and coach', so the appraisal has evolved into:

- Two-way rather than one-way communication
- A process rather than an event
- A developmental process, although rating performance is still an important element of NHS appraisal.

The formal appraisal provides an opportunity to draw together the threads of a work-based dialogue that should have been ongoing throughout the period under review. Appraisal is not a disciplinary process, nor is it a disciplinary discussion. Existing processes for addressing serious issues about conduct or capability should be used appropriately. Neither is appraisal a discussion you 'save things up for': there should be no surprises in the appraisal discussion.

Benefits of appraisal

Appraisal should bring benefits for the appraisee, the organization and the line manager (*Table 16.1*).

Table 16.1. Benefits of appraisal	
Benefits to the organization	A consistent process for recognizing and managing staff performance
	A source of information for planning and decision making
	A way of analysing and responding to development needs
	Improved communication and staff motivation
Benefits to the line manager	A framework for sharing feedback, discussing performance and fixing problems
	A structure for reviewing and aligning the contributions of team members
	Planning future performance through the use of work-based or learning objectives
	Feedback on own management style and approach
Benefits to the appraisee	Constructive feedback including praise and 'improvement focussed' criticism
	A chance to focus on developing his/her individual peformance
	Having a voice in the team's planning
	Having an opportunity to raise problems, barriers and obstacles
	Coming away with a clear set of work and personal development objectives, a better understanding of standards and requirements, and an action plan for future development

The NHS appraisal scheme for doctors

Appraisal aims to 'give doctors feedback on their past performance, to chart their continuing progress and to identify development needs' (Department of Health, 2007a). The standard NHS appraisal scheme (introduced in 2002) aims to address inconsistencies in earlier local, specialty and organizational schemes. It also embeds performance review into managerial processes following the Bristol and Shipman inquiries and accommodates the increasing complexity of doctors' working practices (Department for Education and Skills, 2001).

While supporting continuing professional development, the NHS system also aims to identify and support poorly or under-performing doctors, although appraisal should not be the main way in which poor performance is identified or addressed. Appraisal should provide early identification of individual performance issues or aspects for development, albeit with the ultimate aim of improving clinical performance and patient care.

Doctors' appraisal is closely linked to revalidation, with both frameworks based around the headings in *Good Medical Practice* (General Medical Council, 2006, 2008). The main elements of appraisal are similar for all doctors, although details differ between trainees, consultants, academic clinicians, non-consultant career grade doctors and GPs. The schemes are continuously being revised with a view to streamlining activities.

The links between NHS appraisal, performance review and revalidation have led to concerns that, despite the Department of Health's emphasis on appraisal being on the appraisee's developmental needs, somehow 'appraisal will root out poorly performing doctors' (Department of Health, 2007a). The NHS scheme's inherent tensions and contradictions relate to unrealistically trying to serve three ends through one process: performance management, an educational emphasis on development, and improvement of quality (Taylor et al, 2002). Performance review, clinical governance and audit should run parallel to the appraisal process, so that issues are identified early and remedies and support set in place. This counteracts the potential for 'dumping' issues relating to poor performance into the appraisal scheme when they should be dealt with by local procedures for under-performance or low competence (Department of Health, 2007b).

Other practical issues include:

- Providing training for appraisers
- Providing time (and funding) for preparation
- Possible overlap and conflicts between trainees' annual workplace appraisals, regular training reviews, panels and workplace-based assessments.

The importance of preparation

Successful appraisal depends on careful preparation, including selecting evidence and completing reflective tasks.

The NHS appraisal scheme requires doctors to complete standard forms and collect information from various sources (patients, colleagues and their own reflections) which provide the basis of the appraisal discussion and the personal development plan. These (and a range of guidance documents) can be found on the Department of Health appraisal site (Department of Health, 2009). The Appraisal Toolkit (Department of Health, 2005) is the official site for completing appraisal paperwork, enabling online sharing of information between appraisee and appraiser and the production of the personal development plan.

Appraisal is a two-way process, and preparation should therefore involve the appraisee as well as the appraiser. Both parties should identify specific examples of good performance and difficulties encountered, review 'on-the-job' feedback received, make time for personal reflection and consider the generic requirements within their current post. The organizational context in which the doctor works may lead to additional preparation, e.g. clinical academics are required to undertake joint academic and clinical appraisal and performance reviews often take place at the same time as appraisal, using the same evidence and process to achieve multiple goals (see Chapter 3). The job description, departmental plans and competency profiles might all provide useful evidence. Appraisees might start to identify topics for the appraisal discussion by listing what they are proud of, major achievements, what (or who) has helped or hindered, and any major difficulties encountered.

The physical and interpersonal environment

An effective appraisal discussion needs to consider both the physical and the interpersonal environment. The physical environment should be:
- Private – being seen threatens privacy as much as being heard
- Quiet – background noise inhibits free-flowing discussion
- Relaxed – but not too relaxed …
- On neutral territory – being in 'your office' may reinforce status issues and make people less likely to feel at ease
- Free from distractions – divert your calls and stop interruptions. Taking, or worse still making, telephone calls during an appraisal is not acceptable. This is valuable time devoted specifically to the appraisee
- Professional but comfortable – sitting either side of a desk can psychologically suggest opposition.

The interpersonal environment has huge influence on the degree to which the job-holder feels free to contribute to discussion. You should be aiming for a 70:30 (appraisee:appraiser) ratio in terms of the conversation. Achieving this requires empathy and rapport. Rapport promotes cooperation, openness and trust and enhances communication. Empathy (being able to see a situation through the other person's eyes) helps establish rapport.

Begin the discussion with a friendly, non-threatening question that shows interest – this helps shake off early nerves and show concern for comfort by considering the layout of the room, having water available and taking a break if the discussion becomes lengthy or 'difficult'.

Structuring and managing the appraisal interview

Exploring past performance is essential, but too long spent discussing past performance may mean there is insufficient time for quality planning. This defeats the purpose of appraisal. As part of the interview preparation, an agenda of the main areas to cover should be agreed. This should allow time for aspects of strong performance to be highlighted, praised and encouraged, and areas needing improvement to be explored neutrally and productively.

The skills of effective feedback include productive praise and constructive criticism (see Chapter 5). Productive praise is intended to support the appraisee, highlighting skills and behaviours for development. It is not simply routine encouragement or to compensate for negative comments. Constructive criticism is given to enable the appraisee to consider improvements to future performance, not to apportion blame.

Feedback needs to be related to specific examples and should be descriptive and illustrative, not judgmental, for example:

'You really need to get yourself organized, it's causing enormous problems for everyone in the team and impacting on patients...'

Such judgmental feedback invites a defensive response which can block consideration of the improvements you would like to see the appraisee achieve.

'Keeping patient records up-to-date is crucial. We recently discussed Dr Andrews' difficulties with a paediatric consultation because you had mislaid two of the test results. How have you been able to improve on this?'

The descriptive approach creates a more objective and productive basis for constructive discussion and planning.

The appraisal discussion needs to be managed, taking each agenda item through to completion in a separate communication cycle (*Figure 16.1*).

Figure 16.1. Communication cycle.

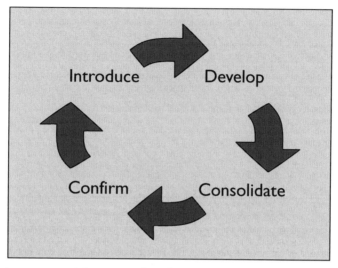

For each item, you might proceed as follows:

- Introduce – with a good open question
- Develop – by listening and asking appropriate probing questions
- Consolidate – by adding observations and feedback, agreeing objectives for future performance or activities for their personal development plan
- Conclude – by briefly summarizing what has been covered and agreed.

Then move on to the next agenda item.

If the appraisee wanders off topic, you can bring the discussion back on track through the 'parking' technique: acknowledging the point, while saying something like 'let's come back to that when we look at teamwork later'. Some flexibility should be retained so that important points additional to the agreed agenda can be addressed.

The key role of self-assessment

Things the appraisee observes, says or decides for him/herself may well have a stronger impact on positive change than your observations. Developing the 'ask-don't-tell habit' Downey (1999) uses open questions to encourage self-appraisal. Compare the following:

Evaluative statement:

'You've got to be sharper and take a lot more care when taking patient histories. Mistakes or areas missed can really jeopardize the chances of an accurate diagnosis.'

Open question:

'Tell me about your use of patient histories as part of diagnosis?'

The latter requires the appraisee to respond with specific examples, e.g. 'well, that's an area where I've run into a few difficulties', you can then ask 'what sort of difficulties?' followed by 'talk me through an example?' This helps the appraisee identify solutions and improvements for him/herself. Your role is to add appropriate observations and help the appraisee refine his/her suggestions.

Skilful questioning

Skilful questioning is the key to successful appraisals. The funnel technique (*Figure 16.2*) is a useful visual reference for questioning skills.

At the mouth of the funnel, begin with an 'open' question which gives the appraisee wide scope in which to respond. You may need to repeat or rephrase this question to allow more thinking time. As the funnel narrows,

Figure 16.2. The 'funnel' technique.

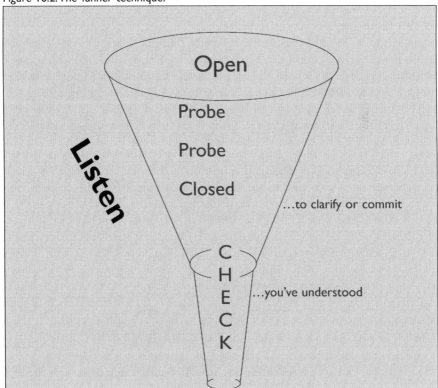

probing questions draw out further specific information to complete the picture. Closed questions are used to check or confirm specific pieces of information, or to get the appraisee to commit to a point more precisely. At the bottom of the funnel, a short paraphrased summary clarifies and checks understanding of the main points.

A question sequence might be:

- 'Tell me how you went about...?' open
- 'How did you prepare?' open (secondary)
- 'What was your starting point?' probe
- 'So, what happened next?' probe
- 'Who else was involved?' probe
- 'And how did they respond?' probe
- 'What were your thoughts at that stage?' probe
- 'What were the main outcomes?' probe
- 'So, that took a total of 6 weeks?' closed – clarifying
- 'Was it your idea or someone else's?' closed – clarifying
- 'And the patient made a full recovery?' closed – clarifying
- 'So, let me see if I've followed you...' checking – summary.

Active listening

Running along the side of the funnel is the word 'listen'. It can be challenging to stay focused and really listen, particularly in a formal discussion such as appraisal. You may be thinking ahead to what your next question is going to be, waiting to speak instead of listening. 'Active listening' helps here, responding through eye contact, nodding, small facial expressions and the occasional echoing of words.

The acronym LISTEN summarizes the features of active listening:

L = Look interested – get interested
I = Involve yourself by responding
S = Stay on target
T = Test your understanding
E = Evaluate the message
N = Neutralize your feelings.

Work and personal development objectives

One output from appraisal is the personal development plan, comprising carefully tailored clinical, educational and personal development objectives which include 'work objectives' focusing on the appraisee's agreed and expected 'contribution' to the team goals and 'personal development objectives' based on areas of agreed 'improvement' in job performance. Objectives should incorporate three development areas:

1. Remedy – to address poor performance
2. Consolidation – to maintain and push forward an 'acceptable' level of performance
3. Growth and diversification – to encourage and 'stretch' individuals who exceed normal performance standards.

The SMART (specific, measurable, agreed/achievable, realistic and timebound) acronym provides a valuable aide-memoire for writing good, effective objectives. In appraisal, three areas are particularly important:

1. Be specific – be clear about the improvement area the objective is focused upon – ambiguity makes an objective very difficult to review at a later stage
2. Make it measurable – be clear about how the improvement will be evaluated at some future point – how will we know it has been achieved?
3. Ensure it is agreed (or at least accepted) – working from agreement that the improvement is desirable is the best way of approaching writing objectives.

The appraisal needs to include regular review of objectives in response to events and changing circumstances.

Conclusions

Done well, appraisal can be very valuable; done badly it can be superficial, discouraging and demotivating. Being clear about what appraisals are for, preparing carefully, and using a good 'coaching' style with an emphasis on self-assessment are keys to successful appraisal. The outcomes of an effective appraisal discussion are praise for work well done, with clear examples that enable the appraisee to go on doing them well or better, constructive criticism of areas requiring improvement with an agreed plan of objectives, goals and support that will provide a firm basis for development and a well-motivated, involved and committed team member who has a clear sense of support and direction.

KEY POINTS

- The aim of appraisal is to improve future clinical, managerial and educational performance while reviewing past performance.
- Appraisal is a positive, developmental, structured process not a one-off event, disciplinary process or disciplinary discussion.
- Appraisal is a two-way process and good, early preparation by both parties is essential.
- Many of the skills underlying effective feedback and supervision are useful for the appraisal interview.
- A poor appraisal can be discouraging and demotivating.
- A wealth of information is available to support appraisees and appraisers engaging in the NHS appraisal scheme.

References

Department for Education and Skills (2001) *A review of appraisal, disciplinary and reporting arrangements for senior NHS and university staff with academic and clinical duties*. DfES, London

Department of Health (2005) The Appraisal Toolkit. www.dh.gov.uk/en/ Managingyourorganisation/Humanresourcesandtraining/EducationTraining andDevelopment/Appraisals/DH_4080426 (accessed 24 April 2009)

Department of Health (2007a) Appraisal questions and answers. www.dh.gov.uk/en/ Managingyourorganisation/Human resourcesandtraining/EducationTrainingand Development/Appraisals/index.htm (accessed 24 April 2009)

Department of Health (2007b) Appraisals: sharing best practice. www. dh.gov.uk/en/Managing yourorganisation/Humanresourcesandtraining/ EducationTrainingandDevelopment/Appraisals/index.htm (accessed 24 April 2009)

Department of Health (2009) Appraisals. www.dh.gov.uk/en/Managingyourorganisation/ Humanresourcesandtraining/EducationTraining andDevelopment/Appraisals/index.htm (accessed 24 April 2009)

Downey M (1999) *Effective Coaching*. Orion Business Books, London

General Medical Council (2006) *Good Medical Practice*. www.gmc-uk.org/guidance/good_ medical_practice/index.asp (accessed 24 April 2009)

General Medical Council (2008) *Draft Framework for Appraisal and Assessment derived from Good Medical Practice*. www.gmc-uk.org/doctors/licensing/docs/Framework_4_3. pdf (accessed 4 May 2009)

Taylor CM, Wall DW, Taylor CL (2002) Appraisal of doctors: problems with terminology and a philosophical tension. *Med Educ* **36**(7): 667–71

CHAPTER 17

Careers support

Caroline Elton

In the wake of the Modernising Medical Careers reforms, the issue of careers support has risen up the medical education agenda. This chapter looks at best practice in providing careers support to junior doctors and considers how to advise trainees whose career plans you believe to be unrealistic.

This chapter looks at how best to support trainee doctors with their career planning. It begins with a consideration of why trainee doctors need careers support, and who is best placed to provide it. Next, the importance of having a structured approach to careers support is explained and the four-stage model (self assessment, career exploration, decision making, plan implementation) is outlined in some detail. The chapter concludes with some suggestions about how best to approach the task of supporting a trainee whose career plans may be unrealistic.

The need for careers support

Before the introduction of *Modernising Medical Careers*, studies demonstrated that there were deficiencies in both the quality and the quantity of careers support within medicine (Lambert et al, 2000; Jackson et al, 2003; Lambert and Goldacre, 2007). Yet with the introduction of the *Modernising Medical Careers* system in August 2005, the need for appropriate careers support has intensified as junior doctors are now required to make major career decisions 18 months after finishing their undergraduate training. This is a significant shift in the timeline of medical career planning as before *Modernising Medical Careers*, even 3 years after leaving medical school, the majority of junior doctors did not regard their career choices as definitive (Goldacre et al, 2004).

Who should provide careers support?

A NICEC (National Institute for Careers Education and Counselling) study of medical students and junior doctors found that the most frequent source of careers advice was senior doctors (Jackson et al, 2003). The guidelines for both the foundation (NHS Foundation Programme, 2009) and post-foundation (Department of Health, 2008) training programmes state that all trainees should receive careers support from educational supervisors. Trainees with more complex career difficulties may need additional careers support from other educational faculty at trust level (e.g. foundation programme training directors, directors of medical education), or from deanery or university careers professionals.

The importance of a framework

In a large scale study of work-based career discussions, Hirsh et al (2001) found that if the providers and recipients of careers support shared a common framework, the recipients found the discussions more useful. Within a higher education careers context, the four-stage model of careers support below is commonly used. This is also the model used in the national medical careers website (www.medicalcareers.nhs.uk):

1. Self assessment
2. Career exploration
3. Decision making
4. Plan implementation.

Using this four-stage framework (and sharing it with trainees) facilitates a systematic approach to providing careers support. In the first session with a new trainee it is good practice to check his/her understanding of the framework and to find out where the trainee thinks he/she is in the overall process of career planning.

Helping a student or trainee with Stage 1: Self-assessment

Students or trainees may consider a number of different aspects as part of the self-assessment phase. As a bare minimum, supervisors should encourage the medical student or trainee to reflect on:

- Achievements, skills and interests
- Aspects of work that he/she finds particularly stressful
- Work values.

Some medical schools and deaneries provide career planning workshops for students or trainees with opportunities to complete various self-assessment tasks. The national medical careers website (www.medicalcareers.nhs.uk) also contains relevant self-assessment exercises. If the learner brings the completed self-assessment exercises to a supervision session, these can be used as a starting point for a career planning discussion.

The list below gives examples of the sorts of questions that a supervisor could pose about a trainee's achievements, skills and interests:

- Through analysing specific achievements of which you feel particularly proud, what key skills did you identify?
- Of these skills, which are you most interested in using at work?
- How does your list of key skills tally with any relevant assessments that have been carried out at medical school, or as part of the foundation programme?
- Are there any key skills that you are not currently using at work that you would like to be able to use, in order to find work more satisfying?

Similar questions can be posed to a trainee to explore other self-assessment exercises that he/she may have carried out, e.g. on work values or on aspects of work that he/she finds particularly stressful.

The role of psychometric testing

Some trainees struggle with self-assessment exercises or, having completed them, have difficulty using the results to identify possible appropriate career options. For these trainees, completing a personality assessment (such as the Myers–Briggs Type Indicator; Myers and McCaulley, 1985) or an interest inventory such as the Sci59 Specialty Choice Inventory (Gale and Grant, 2002) can be useful.

However, Borges and Savickas (2002), in a comprehensive review of the literature on personality tests and medical specialties, concluded that there is more variation in personality traits within medical specialties than between them and more than one medical specialty fits the personality of any particular medical student. They therefore recommend that completing personality tests should be used as a way of increasing self-knowledge, rather than as a diagnostic process to 'match' a particular personality to a particular specialty.

Similarly, if a student or trainee decides to complete the Sci59 inventory, the results should be regarded as a list of possible careers that he/she might want to explore further, rather than as a 'diagnosis' of specialties that will definitely suit that particular individual.

Helping a student or trainee with Stage 2: Career exploration

The key task for the educational supervisor is to encourage the trainee to conduct a thorough exploration of different career options that interest him/her before any final decisions are made. At the outset, it can be helpful to highlight that:

- Career exploration takes time so the student or trainee needs to ensure that this stage is not rushed
- Career exploration does not take place in a vacuum. Instead, the results of the self-assessment phase inform the particular questions that each student or trainee should research when exploring career options
- Even if the trainee thinks he/she knows what he/she wants to do post-foundation, he/she still needs to go through the career exploration phase. This is because being able to articulate his/her particular skills, abilities and interests from stage 1, and then match this list systematically to the demands of a particular specialty (Stage 2), forms the basis of providing solid answers on written application forms or at interview.

Sources of information

The national medical careers website (www.medicalcareers.nhs.uk) can form the starting point of career exploration as it contains comprehensive information on every specialty. In addition, learners should look at the websites of any relevant deaneries and Royal Colleges, as well as the archive of useful articles at BMJ Careers (www.bmjcareers.com). The Modernising Medical Careers website (www.mmc.nhs.uk) contains information about how competitive the different specialties were in the previous application round.

Supervisors can also encourage trainees to explore key journals in specialty areas that they are considering. Although many of the articles may be too specialized, a trainee can ask him-/herself whether he/she is gripped and intrigued by the articles, or whether the content leaves him/her somewhat cold.

Tasters

Undoubtedly the best way to find out if you are suited to a particular career option is to try it out. Some trainees can do this, as they will be applying for an option that they worked in during a foundation placement. If this was not possible (either because there are no foundation placements in that specialty, or because the trainee did not succeed in getting that particular placement) then they should arrange a 'taster' week. Trainees need to avoid being in the position where they are applying post-foundation for a specialty in which they have had neither a placement nor a taster.

Helping a trainee with Stage 3: Career decision making

When helping a trainee with the process of career decision making, one approach is to ask the trainee about a previous important decision that he/she feels (in retrospect) worked out well, not necessarily a career decision. Ask the trainee what made it a good decision and how he/she went about reaching that particular decision. The supervisor can then ask the trainee if there are any decisions that he/she feels (in retrospect) did not work out so well. What can the trainee learn from this example about how not to make an important decision in future?

To support trainees with the content of their career decision making, the ROADS acronym (Elton and Reid, 2007) can be used to structure the discussion through posing the following questions:

Realistic:	Are you being realistic about yourself and about the demands of the job?
Opportunities:	Have you considered seriously all the opportunities available?
Anchors:	Have you built in the things that provide support in your life?
Development:	Do your choices fully develop your potential?
Stress:	Have you considered the aspects of work that create particular stresses for you?

A plan and a back-up

Borges et al (2004) indicated that there is no one perfect specialty choice for each person. Students or trainees should be helped to understand how choosing different specialties would construct satisfying and successful careers. It is sound practice to encourage trainees to have a back-up plan (preferably with a less competitive specialty), that they would also be happy to pursue if they are not successful with their first choice.

Trainees who are seriously considering leaving medicine

The educational supervisor's first task is to explore whether there are some educational difficulties in the trainee's current placement or current mental or physical health issues that are contributing to the situation. In these situations a supervisor would need to liaise with senior educational faculty who had responsibility for that particular training programme. But if it seems that lack of educational support or health problems are not the issue, then the trainee should be advised to seek more specialist careers support from senior educational faculty at the trust, or from careers providers at the university or deanery.

Helping a trainee with Stage 4: Plan implementation

The role of the supervisor at this point is to encourage the trainee to give adequate attention to completing application forms and/or CVs and preparing for the interview or selection centre process.

Issues that a supervisor might discuss with the trainee include:

- The practicalities of the application process: how many applications can be submitted and the closing dates.
- Being suitably prepared before the application process goes 'live'. Time scales for the opening and closing of a given specialty application can be very short. Trainees need to look at the previous year's person specification in advance and choose relevant examples from their portfolio that match the different elements of the person specification. When the application process starts for real, all the trainee needs to do is check whether there are any significant changes between the new person specification and the previous one.
- Checking and double checking all forms and CVs. Spelling or grammatical mistakes give a sloppy impression.
- Plagiarism. The trainee needs to look at the advice that has been given on this issue and then adhere to it.

Interview preparation

Different specialties use different selection processes for post-foundation specialty recruitment. Specific information is available on the Modernising Medical Careers and Royal College websites. If a trainee is applying for a specialty that uses formal interviews, he/she should think through the sorts of questions that he/she is likely to be asked and prepare strong answers to them. The trainee should also know his/her portfolio inside out, and be able to use it to give specific examples of key skills and abilities as well as examples of areas in which he/she was initially weaker, and what he/she did to improve performance in these areas.

A trainee whose career plans may be unrealistic

In this situation, the educational supervisor should pose challenging questions to the trainee, such as:

- What does the trainee see as his/her key strengths?
- How does this self-assessment of his/her key strengths tie in with some of the assessment evidence in his/her portfolio?
- In which areas has he/she been assessed as being less strong? Are any of these areas important in terms of demonstrating suitability for the specialty of interest?
- Has the trainee researched the likely competitiveness for the specialty of interest?
- What are his/her thoughts on the fact that he/she is interested in a particularly competitive specialty but he/she has not been assessed as being particularly strong in some of the key competences?

If a trainee persists in holding onto his/her career aspirations, despite a full discussion of these sorts of issues with his/her supervisor, he/she could be offered an additional careers support session with a senior consultant in his/her specialty of interest, or with a specialist careers adviser.

While educational supervisors have to behave responsibly to the trainee, they are not responsible for the trainee's career decisions. So if a particular trainee wants to ignore the facts about how competitive it is to succeed in his/her chosen pathway, then ultimately that is his/her decision. The educational supervisor's role is to ensure that the relevant issues have been raised in a clear, yet supportive way. It is not always possible to stop some people from making poor career decisions (Kidd, 2006).

Career planning and lifelong learning

Finally it needs to be emphasized that career decision making does not end once the trainee has chosen his/her specialty. Doctors need to make career decisions throughout the whole of their career, e.g. sub-specialty choices, the type of hospital or GP practice they want to work in or additional responsibilities they want to pursue. That career planning is a lifelong task is specifically mentioned in the operational framework of the Foundation Programme (NHS Foundation Programme, 2009) and also accords with contemporary approaches to careers support (Krieshok et al, 2009).

Conclusions

One of the effects of the Modernising Medical Careers reforms of postgraduate medical education is that trainees have to make significant career decisions 18 months after leaving medical school. The independent inquiry into Modernising Medical Careers recognized the importance of improving the quality and quantity of careers support from medical school onwards (Tooke, 2008). While educational supervisors will be the primary source of careers support, specialist services should also be made available at university or deanery level. This chapter has highlighted the importance of the provider of the careers support adopting a structured approach to career planning, and sharing this overall four-stage framework with the trainees. In this way, trainees will be encouraged to approach the task of career planning systematically and thoroughly. But it is equally important to emphasize that career planning does not cease when a trainee has chosen his/her specialty pathway. Instead, the acquisition of the career planning skills needed to navigate a path through the four stages of the career framework is an essential aspect of a trainee's overall professional development.

KEY POINTS

- The effectiveness of careers support is enhanced if both the recipient and provider work from a shared framework.
- The four-stage model (self-assessment, career exploration, decision making, plan implementation) provides an appropriate framework for the provision of careers support.
- It is important to encourage the student or trainee to spend sufficient time on each of the four stages.
- Clinical faculty with educational responsibilities should also recognize when it may be appropriate to refer a particular student or trainee for specialist careers support.
- Acquiring key career planning skills is not only necessary for specialty choice, but is an essential component of ongoing professional development.

References

Borges NJ, Savickas ML (2002) Personality and medical specialty choice: a literature review and integration. *J Career Assess* **10:** 362–80

Borges NJ, Savickas ML, Jones BJ (2004) Holland's theory applied to medical specialty choice. *J Career Assess* **12:** 188–206

Department of Health (2008) *A Reference Guide for Postgraduate Specialty Training in the UK ('Gold Guide')*. Department of Health, London

Elton C, Reid J (2007) *The ROADS to Success: A practical approach to career planning for medical students, foundation trainees (and their supervisors)*. Postgraduate Deanery for Kent Surrey and Sussex, London

Gale R, Grant J (2002) Sci45: the development of a specialty choice inventory. *Med Educ* **36:** 659–66

Goldacre MJ, Turner G, Lambert TW (2004) Variation by medical school in career choices of UK graduates of 1999 and 2000. *Med Educ* **38:** 249–58

Hirsh W, Jackson C, Kidd J (2001) *Straight Talking: Effective Career Discussions at Work*. National Institute for Careers Education and Counselling, Cambridge

Jackson C, Hirsh W, Kidd J (2003) *Informing Choices. The need for career advice in medical training*. National Institute for Careers Education and Counselling, Cambridge

Kidd JM (2006) *Understanding Career Counselling: Theory, Research and Practice*. Sage, London

Krieshok TS, Black MD, McKay RA (2009) Career decision making: the limits of rationality and the abundance of non-conscious processes. *J Voc Behav* (in press) doi:10.1016/j.jvb.2009.04.006

Lambert TW, Goldacre MJ (2007) Views of doctors in training on the importance and availability of career advice in UK medicine. *Med Educ* **41:** 460–6

Lambert TW, Goldacre MJ, Evans J (2000) Views of junior doctors about their work: survey of qualifiers of 1993 and 1996 from United Kingdom Medical Schools. *Med Educ* **34:** 348–54

Myers IB, McCaulley M (1985) *Manual: a guide to the use of the Myers-Briggs Type Indicator*. Consulting Psychologists Press, New York

NHS Foundation Programme (2009) *Operational Framework for Foundation Training, NHS Foundation Programme*. www.foundationprogramme.nhs.uk/pages/home/key-documents (accessed 21 September 2009)

Tooke J (2008) *Aspiring to Excellence: Final Report of the Independent Inquiry into Modernising Medical Careers*. Universities UK, London (www.mmcinquiry.org.uk) (accessed 21 September 2009)

CHAPTER 18

Mentoring

Rebecca Viney and Judy McKimm

Many clinical teachers and supervisors may be required to act as a mentor for a colleague, either informally or as part of a formal scheme. The skills required of an effective mentor are similar to those of a coach, involving career advice, goal setting and support, and can be learned and applied in a range of work-based situations.

This chapter sets out the principles of mentoring, what mentoring is and what it is not. It considers the benefits to mentors, mentees and organizations in different contexts and the factors underpinning successful mentoring schemes. It outlines the typical topics brought to mentoring, possible traps that mentors can fall into and provides some examples of questions useful for mentoring conversations.

What is mentoring?

Mentoring is difficult to define. Many different definitions abound, but three useful ones are:

- 'Guiding another individual in the development and re-examination of their own ideas, learning and personal and professional development' (Standing Committee on Postgraduate Medical and Dental Education, 1998)
- 'Off line help by one person to another in making significant transitions in knowledge, work or thinking' (Megginson and Clutterbuck, 1995)
- 'Someone who helps another person to become what that person aspires to be' (Applebaum et al, 1994).

Other research defines mentoring based on what it is not, for example Connor and Pokora (2007) contrast mentoring and coaching with patronage and therapy (*Table 18.1*).

Table 18.1. Patronage and therapy: why is mentoring different?

Patronage	Mentoring and coaching	Therapy
Career advancement	Problems and opportunities	Personal problems and difficulties
Career-related	Work- or career-related	Issues may be deeply personal and/or unrelated to work
Patron unlikely to be trained	Coach/mentor uses skills and framework	Therapist is a qualified practitioner
Boundaries less important, may be intentional overlap	Coach/mentor agrees boundaries	Therapist operates strict boundaries
May be same profession/field	Coach/mentor may be internal or external	Therapist is outside organization
Patron opens doors	Emphasis is on learning and development	Therapist helps to resolve problems
Patron is senior	Coach/mentor may be senior, colleague, junior or development	Therapist is impartial and independent
Patron may not expect feedback on relationship	Feedback is part of the learning relationship	Amount and use of feed back depends on thera-peutic approach

Mentoring is very complex. It varies from one situation to another, and is interpreted in different ways by different people, but it is important that the purpose and intentions of mentoring in each particular context are made explicit. Others define mentoring by comparing it with counselling, coaching, appraisal and clinical supervision (*Table 18.2*).

Coaching and mentoring focus on personal, professional and career development. Coaching tends to be shorter term and task orientated and mentoring is more usually longer but there is a great deal of overlap between coaching and mentoring skills. *Figure 18.1* shows the differences in terms of focus and issues.

Table 18.2. Mentoring and other support mechanisms

Coaching	Coaching is a method of developing an individual's capabilities in order to facilitate the achievement of personal and organizational success
	It focuses on skills and performance, the agenda is set by or with the coach, typically a line manager role
Mentoring	Mentoring focuses on capability and potential, it works best if off-line. The agenda is entirely set by the learner. It typically assists with managing job transition, career choices and career development
	There are benefits to the individual, the organization and to patient care
Counselling	A qualified professional helps resolve personal issues which may or may not be work related. The problem may be around a relationship or health issue
	The professional is impartial and has firm boundaries
Appraisal	Appraisal should be a vibrant educational process. It is a means of preparing the ground for enhancing personal development and contributes to partnership between an individual and the employing organization (Conlon, 2003)
Clinical supervision	Supervision has been defined in many ways, but is essentially a conversation between professionals aimed at promoting learning, reflective practice and improving patient safety and the quality of patient care (see Chapter 6)

Figure 18.1. Mentoring, counselling, coaching and job planning: what are the differences?

	Private issues		
Person focus	**Counselling**	**Coaching**	**Task focus**
	Mentoring	**Job planning**	
	Job issues		

What are the benefits to individuals, organizations and patients?

The benefits of mentoring for mentees, mentors, patients and the host organization have been widely documented (*Table 18.3*). Benefits for individuals include improved motivation, job satisfaction and problem solving. Garvey and Garrett-Harris (2005) found that the main four benefits of mentoring to mentees were:

1. Improved performance and productivity
2. Career opportunity and advancement
3. Improved knowledge and skills
4. Greater confidence and wellbeing.

Table 18.3. The benefits of mentoring	
Motivation	Improved job satisfaction and motivation
	Improved commitment to employing organization
	Improved career progression
	Potential rejuvenation of longer serving staff
Performance	Enhanced achievement of targets
	Increased productivity
	Reduced complaints
Policy implementation	Improved staff retention
	Improved implementation of diversity policy
	Better management of 'talent'
	Aids development of empowerment policies
Knowledge and skills benefit	Faster learning
	Widens experience
	Developing new knowledge and skills
	Supporting innovation
Managing change	Support for culture change
	Support for reorganization and restructuring
	Support for people in new roles and new jobs
	Helps develop a positive attitude to change
Succession planning	Leadership skills
	Improved succession planning, confidence and wellbeing in change situations
	Adapted from Garvey and Garrett-Harris (2005)

Benefits for organizations include improved team functioning, promotion of cultural diversity, quality enhancement and better management of conflict between colleagues and patients.

What are typical topics in medical mentoring?

Medical mentoring is usually about maximizing potential. Some doctors are already very good but want to be the best. They need help to manage their talent and develop leadership skills, and a coaching style may be most appropriate for this group. Some doctors are in transition and want to achieve a better work–life balance or have major decisions to make. The third, much smaller, group comprises those doctors who are in difficulty and seek outside support to help them tackle and survive adversity. So the breadth of mentoring covers:

- Growing talent
- Developing leadership skills
- Managing change
- Career decisions
- Achieving work–life balance
- Developing resilience in times of adversity.

It is important that the mentor is well networked and knows how to access other sources of help for the mentee, such as careers information, counselling, psychotherapy or medical help.

What factors lead to a successful mentoring scheme?

In order to facilitate mentoring within organizations (such as NHS trusts, primary care trusts, postgraduate deaneries or Royal Colleges) and encourage successful outcomes, certain environmental conditions must prevail and an enabling framework must be established.

Conway (1994) suggests that the business case for a facilitated mentoring scheme must be clearly articulated and senior management must firmly believe in the concept and demonstrate this commitment. The mechanics, structures and support for the key people must be in place and clear to all concerned. When making out the business case for a facilitated mentoring scheme the questions in *Table 18.4* need to be explored.

Facilitated mentoring schemes have more successful outcomes when the mentoring is entirely voluntary, confidentiality is ensured and the process is promoted as a valuable form of personal and professional development. Mentors themselves benefit from substantive training, with assessment and

Table 18.4. Establishing a mentoring scheme

Why do we need a mentoring programme?	What are the aims for the programme?
	What do we hope to achieve?
Is mentoring consonant with our organisational structures and values?	Is mentoring already happening?
	Has it been tried before?
Who will be involved – mentors/mentees?	
Who will 'run' the initiative?	
What problems do we anticipate?	
Who will our mentors be?	Do we need to produce a mentor profile?
	How will we select them?
Who is to be mentored?	Why?
	What is the aim for the group of mentees and for individuals?
	How will they be selected?
How will mentors and mentees be matched and paired?	
What resources are required and available?	
What briefing and training will be required by:	mentees?
	other stakeholders?
How will mentors be	supported?
	rewarded?
When and how will the mentoring programme be monitored and evaluated? And by whom?	

ongoing education, support and supervision. The schemes that thrive have commitment from the top, with adequate time, funds and space to ensure a quality service. Monitoring and evaluation of feedback from all stakeholders should be continuous. The mentoring itself should be time limited, have a contractual arrangement, a no-blame opt-out clause, and be focused with objectives. Successful schemes usually have a lead who is able to promote, manage and be flexible. Good communication and marketing to the entire organization and potential participants is also an important factor.

How to create a successful scheme

- Voluntary participation
- Visible participation and support by senior members

- Trained mentors with ongoing support
- A clear matching policy, preferably with choice
- Clear ground rules and an ethical code of practice
- The agenda belongs to the mentee.

Types of mentoring in medicine

Mentoring is only one form of support. Individuals may be supported in other ways, e.g. by colleagues (peer support), line managers, counsellors, tutors or teachers and groups, e.g. action learning sets or work teams, friends or parents. Individuals may have a mix of support, for a number of reasons varying over time, including more than one mentor. The traditional form of mentoring is one-to-one mentoring but there are other models such as co-mentoring, peer mentoring or group mentoring. Mentoring can also be mentee-initiated and can happen informally when an individual seeks advice and support from another individual. Often people do not recognize that they have a mentor or have been mentoring. This kind of mentoring may occur within or outside an organization.

Principles underpinning good mentoring

A useful set of values and principles that underpin good mentoring are listed in *Figure 18.2*.

What are the characteristics of a good mentor?

Good mentors listen with empathy, share experiences, form mutual learning friendships, enable the development of insight through reflection, act as a sounding board and encourage mentees.

Good mentors sometimes use coaching and counselling behaviours, challenge assumptions, act as role models and open doors as sponsors. However, good mentors never discipline, condemn, appraise formally, assess formally or supervise.

What skills do the mentee and mentor need?

The mentee needs to want to grow and change and should not be referred to mentoring by a third party: to be successful the mentoring must be a voluntary process. The mentor, who should ideally be trained, should be

Figure 18.2. Values and principles underpinning mentoring.

The mentoring process is underpinned by the following values and principles:
Recognizing that people are okay (Hay, 1995)
Realizing that people can change and want to grow (Hay, 1995)
Understanding how people learn
Recognizing individual differences
Empowering through personal and professional development
Encouraging capability
Developing competence
Encouraging collaboration not competition
Encouraging scholarship and a sense of enquiry
Searching for new ideas, theories and knowledge
Equal opportunities in the organization
Reflecting on past experiences as a key to understanding
Looking forward (reflexion) and developing the ability to transfer learning and apply it in new situations
Realizing that we can create our own meaning of mentoring (Hay, 1995)

assessed and supported in his/her role, with a clear ethical code of practice and equal opportunity training.

Megginson et al (2006) define the basic competencies that mentors and mentees need as:

- Communication skills to articulate problems and ideas
- Being able to listen and to challenge constructively
- The ability to be honest with oneself and the other partner and to reflect upon what is being said, both at the time and subsequently
- A capacity for empathy.

And Brigden (2000) suggests that mentees require that their mentor:

- Knows what he/she is talking about
- Is not intimidating, but is easy to approach
- Is interested in the mentee personally, and displays genuine concern
- Provides subtle guidance, but ensures the mentee makes decisions
- Actually questions the mentee
- Will debate and challenge the mentee
- Will give honest answers
- Does not blame, stays neutral
- Is enabling, caring, open and facilitative
- Gives constructive and positive feedback.

What makes mentoring work?

The success of mentoring is in the establishment of an effective relationship, based upon mutual respect, honesty and understanding. The mentor doesn't necessarily have to be someone more senior in the organization, but rather needs to have the motivation and training to support the mentee in his/her development. Other qualities of mentors that can enrich the mentoring relationship include a varied career and life experience, a wide professional network and commitment to their own professional development. The mentor needs to have 'something' (a quality, skill or experience) that mentees see as being helpful in their personal or professional life.

Some powerful mentoring questions

The powerful questions of mentoring are derived from motivational interviews, solution-focused coaching and positive psychology. Here is a small selection. They are best used after training as there are a number of traps that you can fall into without guidance. But you might try these out in certain situations and see the difference between advice giving and empowering the mentee.

Goal setting

What do you want?
> *Or*

What should we discuss in this meeting so that the conversation will be useful?

Orientation and motivation

What will that get you?
> *Or*

How will you know that you have achieved it, what will you notice?

Using previous experiences

Have you ever achieved something like this before? How did you do it on that occasion?
> *Or*

Have you ever achieved something like this before? And how will you do it on this occasion?

Action

What would be the first step that you could take to achieve your aims?
   Or
What step will you take? And by when?

Notice that in the second version of the question the future is visualized by the word 'will', so that the mentee sees the current issue being resolved. His/her visualization of this is a first step towards change.

Traps for medical mentors

Doctors are expert at diagnosis, problem solving and advising patients. It is difficult sometimes for the doctor mentor to remember that he/she is not mentoring a patient and that the mentee is whole, capable and resourceful. Doctors may find it difficult not to give advice and even solve the problem for the mentee. Instead the mentor should help the mentee to weigh up situations, through a process of reflection, questions, challenge and feedback allowing the mentee to come to a decision him-/herself. It is crucial to remember that in any mentoring relationship it is the mentee who drives the agenda, not the mentor. Therefore doctor-mentors must refrain from offering advice which may be hard to do, especially as mentees will often ask for advice if they have not had the opportunity to experience the powerful questions of a trained mentor. *Table 18.5* lists what Clutterbuck (1991) (in a 'tongue in cheek' way) describes as the 12 habits of an ineffective mentor.

Conclusions

Mentoring is a rare opportunity to achieve increased effectiveness and change. The mentor's role is to be supportive in an active way which means that the mentor is not just a sympathetic listener, but will prompt and question the mentee through a structured process. However, mentoring has a role not only for the individual doctor but can also transform professional culture when it forms part of an internal, non-hierarchical supportive network that is committed to facilitating personal and professional development. In the words of Mahatma Ghandi: 'real education consists of drawing the best out of yourself.'

Table 18.5. What not to do: twelve habits of an ineffective mentor

1. Start from the point of view that you – from your vast experience and broader perspective – know better than the mentee what's in his or her best interest

2. Be determined to share your wisdom with them – whether they want it or not; remind them frequently how much they have still to learn

3. Decide what you and the mentee will talk about and when; change dates and themes frequently to prevent complacency sneaking in

4. Do most of the talking; check frequently that they are paying attention

5. Make sure that they understand how trivial their concerns are compared to the weighty issues you have to issue with

6. Remind the mentee how fortunate he/she is to have your undivided attention

7. Neither show, nor admit any personal weaknesses. Expect to be their role model in all aspects of career development and personal values

8. Never ask them what they should expect of you – how would they know anyway?

9. Demonstrate how important and well connected you are by sharing confidential information they don't need (or want) to know

10. Discourage any signs of levity or humour – this is a serious business and should be treated as such

11. Take them to task when they don't follow your advice

12. Never, ever admit that this could be a learning experience for both of you

From Clutterbuck (1991)

KEY POINTS

- Mentoring is about releasing potential and must follow the mentee's agenda.
- Standards and qualifications in mentoring are being developed.
- Ethical guidelines should be in place.
- Confidentiality is paramount.
- Evaluation should be a continual, ongoing process.

References

Applebaum SH, Ritchie S, Shapiro BT (1994) Mentoring revisited: an organizational behaviour construct. *International Journal of Career Management* **6**: 3–10

Brigden D (2000) Mentoring: a powerful and cost effective method of encouraging development. *Mersey Deanery Educational Update* 7

Clutterbuck D (1991) *Everyone needs a mentor: fostering talent at work.* Institute of Personnel and Development, London

Conlon M (2003) Appraisal: the catalyst of personal development. *BMJ* **327**: 389–91

Connor M, Pokora J (2007) *Coaching and Mentoring at Work: Developing Effective Practice.* Open University Press, Milton Keynes

Conway C (1994) *Mentoring Managers in Organisations - A Study of Mentoring and its Application to Organisations with Case Studies.* Ashridge Research Group, Ashridge

Garvey B, Garrett-Harris R (2005) The Benefits of Mentoring: A Literature Review, A Report for East mentors Forum. The Coaœching and Mentoring Research Unit, Sheffield Hallam University, Sheffield

Hay J (1995) *Transformational Mentoring.* McGraw Hill, New York

Megginson D, Clutterbuck D (1995) *Mentoring in Action: a practical guide for managers.* Kogan Page, London

Megginson D, Clutterbuck D, Garvey B, Stokes P, Garrett-Harris R (2006) *Mentoring in Action - a practical guide.* Kogan Page, London

Standing Committee on Postgraduate Medical and Dental Education (1998) *Supporting Doctors and Dentists at Work: An Enquiry into Mentoring.* Standing Committee on Postgraduate Medical and Dental Education, London

CHAPTER 19

Managing poor performance

Howard Borkett-Jones and Clare Morris

Trainees may encounter a range of difficulties during their training period. Supporting a trainee in difficulty can be extremely challenging, yet immensely rewarding.

This chapter considers how a supervisor can make a significant difference to the educational outcome for a struggling trainee. It starts by identifying different types of difficulties and linked 'signs and symptoms'. A range of possible intervention and support strategies are then explored. The chapter emphasizes the role of clinical and educational supervisors in supporting trainees.

Introduction

Supervisors of trainees facing difficulties should make themselves aware of local and regional resources and be able to access and use these appropriately when required (*Table 19.1*). This is seldom a role to undertake single-handedly: deaneries and local education providers can offer expert advice, guidance and support.

Diagnosing difficulties

Supporting a trainee in difficulty starts with recognizing common signs and symptoms, followed by a triage process to help distinguish trainees with difficulties, and those in difficulty from those who may be just 'difficult trainees':

1. Trainees in difficulty – a trainee who is failing to make satisfactory progress overall or has areas of specific difficulty with his/her training
2. Trainees with difficulties of a transient nature who, for a certain period of time, need particular support
3. Trainees who many trainers find 'difficult' (the so-called difficult trainee) because of conduct issues.

Table 19.1. Roles and responsibilities of those involved in training	
Trainee	Holds a contractual relationship with employer which reflects local and national terms and conditions of employment
Employing local education provider	Is responsible for management of performance and disciplinary matters, with support from human resources when needed.
	Should keep deanery advised of any issues arising. Educational and clinical supervisors are likely to be involved in the identfication, management and suport of trainee in difficulty.
	Those with more senior educational roles and responsibilities (e.g. clinical or college tutors, training programme directors, director of medical education and, ultimately, the medical director) may become involved depending on nature and severity of dificulties faced
Deanery	Is responsible for all doctors in training and problems which arise that prevent normal progression. They also quality manage training programmes
General Medical Council	May be involved where there are concerns about fitness to practice
	Adapted from National Association of Clinical Tutors (2008)

It is often easier to manage the first two situations than the third. It is helpful to distinguish problems that arise from current circumstances (*Figure 19.1*) from problems that are related specifically to the personality and behaviour patterns of a trainee. Careful 'diagnosis' will guide your choice of intervention strategy, as discussed later in this article.

Recognizing signs and symptoms

Paice (2006) described seven key early warning signs of a trainee in difficulty, in terms of observed behavioural patterns (*Figure 19.2*). If any early warning signs are observed, a first step is to discuss the behaviour with the trainee, being careful to focus on observable behaviours rather than personal characteristics or traits. This may rapidly identify possible cause(s) of the trainee's difficulty which can be dealt with immediately. Some trainees may readily disclose information to a supervisor who clearly indicates his/her willingness to listen and support. Others may have concerns about revealing information to those whom they perceive to be in a position of power.

Figure 19.1. Common circumstantial problems for trainees.

* Educational challenges, exams, revision
* Anxiety concerning career decisions
* Pressure of work, lack of team support
* Unfamiliarity, inexperience
* Changes in team dynamics
* Personal health problems
* Sickness within the family,
* Personal relationship difficulties
* Cultural isolation, culture shock (e.g. overseas graduates)
* Domestic responsibilities or pressures

Figure 19.2. Seven key early warning signs. Adapted from Paice (2006).

* The 'disappearing act': not answering bleeps, disappearing, lateness, frequent sick leave
* Low work rate: slowness in various aspects of work, poor productivity
* 'Ward rage': bursts of temper
* Rigidity: poor tolerance of ambiguity, inability to compromise, difficulty prioritizing, inappropriate 'whistle blowing'
* 'Bypass syndrome': nurses and others avoid seeking the doctor's help
* Career problems: difficulty with exams and career choice, disillusionment with medicine
* Insight failure: rejection of constructive criticism, defensiveness, counter-challenge

Supporting trainees in difficulty

Trainees in difficulty are those who are not making sufficient progress in training or who are experiencing difficulties with certain elements of training. Failure to progress educationally as a doctor usually relates to a failure in learning within the workplace.

Swanwick (2005) describes the role of the trainer as that of 'structuring experiences, rather than transmitting knowledge', underlining the importance of experiences themselves as the vehicle for learning, rather than the knowledge of the trainer. Trainees in difficulty may need help in identifying the learning opportunities that arise in the workplace and encouragement to value and seize the opportunities for learning that they offer. Supervisors can help in making learning opportunities explicit and encouraging engagement. Trainees in difficulty need more experience rather than less, and the supervisor's role in 'safety netting' is important.

Interventions and strategies

A structured training curriculum and workplace-based assessments can furnish a range of helpful 'diagnostic data' and indicate the type(s) of learning experiences trainees may need to make progress. Personal development plans can help trainees recognize gaps in their experience, skills or knowledge and be used to set goals for future development. The facilitation by the educational supervisor of 'developmental conversations', which highlight ways of addressing areas of difficulty, are vital. Multi-source feedback is particularly useful, with careful interpretation of data to identify areas of underperformance. Trainees who consistently overrate their own performance may be a cause for concern.

Observation of trainees' practice in the workplace, formally or informally, can contextualize behaviour reported by others in the team. For example, direct observation of a consenting procedure may simultaneously give insight into weaknesses in communication skills (behavioural characteristic) and technical understanding (knowledge base). *Table 19.2* summarizes common areas of difficulty and how to approach them.

Creating an environment for learning

Trainees need a 'safe' learning environment in order to learn effectively. Maslow (1943) argued that in order for individuals to achieve self-actualization, i.e. to reach their full potential, a range of basic needs have first to be met. Self esteem, confidence and a sense of safety are prerequisites for the 'higher' activities of learning and problem solving to be realized.

Trainees who face difficulties may well struggle to achieve what they are capable of achieving. The need to attend to the emotional dimensions of learning is evident in these situations. Learning in the workplace is about learning with and from others.

'...we learn to collaborate, influence, negotiate, motivate, and achieve results through our interaction with others, all of which can be highly charged with emotion.' (Turnbull, 2000)

Times of uncertainty and insecurity in new jobs are familiar for most doctors, and trainees face these challenges regularly. It is important to ensure that the workplace culture is one which welcomes trainees as part of a team. Trainees in difficulty may need longer than most to recognize and adopt tacit rules of behaviour. Supervisors should also remember the value of positive emotions in educational experiences and correct approaches to learning which exploit fear and humiliation as key 'motivators' – negative approaches to education have little evidence of their effectiveness.

Table 19.2. Common areas of difficulty and how to approach them

Area of difficulty	Approaches to identification	Possible educational interventions
Practical skills/ procedures	DOPs and observed practice Feedback from colleagues Errors reported	Specific feedback and guidance Purposeful observation by those skilled in the procedure. Simulation Close supervision, opportunities to practice
Communication skills	Mini-CEX multi-source feedback, observation. Feedback from patients, carers, colleagues	Specific feedback and guidance Video recording with self review. Formal training
Clinical reasoning	CBD, clinical teaching (on rounds, in clinic) Over-reliance on investigations Diagnostic errors	Developing knowledge base Use socratic questioning techniques in supervision Case-based discussion with a focus on rationale for choices, with consideration of alternatives Increased clinical exposure and requirement to present cases
Insight into performance MSF, self ratings	Multi-source feedback Self ratings Evidence in feedback (capacity to self evaluate) and supervision sessions	Encourage independent review of performance in all feedback sessions Encourage trainee to self rate assessments before sharing your ratings and discuss differences Develop competence through increased opportunities to practice (being able to recognize a competent performance is a key step to developing insight). Regular feedback
Team working	MSF, feedback from colleagues and observed behaviour	Shadowing team members – develop awareness of their roles and contributions Case-based discussion to explore who else to involve in patient management (and why)

CBD = case-based discussion; DOPS = direct observation of procedural skills; mini-CEX = mini clinical evaluation exercise; MSF = multi-source feedback

Moore and Kuol (2007) identified interest, intense positive affect, humour, fun, enjoyment, enthusiasm, commitment, dedication and compassion in students' recollections of excellent teaching, and noted that a teacher's attributes were invoked more frequently than his/her actions by students when recalling positive learning experiences. They concluded that 'who a teacher is with their students' was more relevant in the recollection of good learning experiences than 'what a teacher does with his/her subject'. Almost certainly this will prove to be true for trainees in difficulty.

Supporting trainees with difficulties

The supervisor's role with the trainee with difficulties may be limited to the recognition of early warning signs and 'referral' to colleagues able to provide specific and/or specialist advice or support. Respect for the supervisory boundary is important – the supervisor is neither the trainee's doctor nor his/her counsellor.

Typical difficulties trainees may face are summarized in *Figure 19.1*.

Health issues

Physical and/or mental health issues (e.g. diabetes, depression, epilepsy) may arise during training or be long-standing, and be disclosed to the employer but not to individual supervisors. Subtle health issues may be difficult to discern, and it is helpful to seek input from a range of sources – medical, senior nursing, clerical and secretarial staff – in order to gain a rounded and balanced picture. Some additional support, changes to duties or time out may be sufficient for the trainee to regain health.

Mental health issues, alcohol and drug misuse are more often not disclosed, but where there is cause for concern and patient care or safety may be compromised, advice should be sought from occupational health and human resources immediately. Certain health difficulties may raise issues concerning fitness to practice: the General Medical Council provides guidance in these cases. Whatever the health issues faced, it is important to ensure that trainees are treated fairly.

Personal issues

Trainees may experience difficulties with personal relationships or may have carer responsibilities which detract from full engagement with training. Human resources colleagues can advise the trainee of rights to carer or parental leave.

Where disruption to training is significant, the deanery may advise on options for time out, flexible training or an extension to the training period.

Career development issues

Recent reform of postgraduate training, and changes in selection procedures have undoubtedly been a cause of anxiety and stress for many trainees. In Chapter 17, Elton gives structured guidance on how to help trainees facing difficult decisions with regards to their careers, and those whose career aspirations appear unrealistic.

Managing 'difficult trainees'

Trainees with personal conduct and performance issues are likely to be in the minority but may occupy a considerable amount of the supervisor's time and energy.

Trainees are employees and, as such, should demonstrate appropriate professional behaviour with patients, carers and colleagues. The General Medical Council (2006) guidance *Good Medical Practice* applies to all UK doctors, including those in training.

In practical terms, it is important to distinguish between issues of improper personal conduct, subject to local employment regulations, and issues of poor professional performance. Matters of improper conduct – e.g. absence without leave, theft, bullying, sexual harassment – apply equally to all employees. If a trainee's behaviour or conduct has been questioned, the director of medical education should advise on how any allegations should be investigated in accordance with local human resources policy. Conduct issues with implications for the future professional work of the trainee should be reported to the deanery after investigation at local level. National policies, General Medical Council regulations and any obligations under law must be respected.

The supervisor should ensure that accurate, contemporaneous, dated and signed records of feedback, supervision and appraisal sessions are kept.

Stress and burnout

> *'Doctors are exposed constantly to risks, including stress, alienation, over-involvement, automatic behaviour, and burnout…. The medical profession has until now been in the paradoxical position of needing as much… [support] …as any other group of clinicians (if not more), but generally getting less.' (Launer, 2006)*

The social implications of pursuing a medical career, as well as the cognitive challenges, need to be considered. Firth-Cozens (2003) emphasized the significant levels of stress among junior doctors – with 28% showing above threshold levels of stress, compared to 18% in the general working population. Differences in perceptions of and responses to stressful circumstances may be indicative of personality predispositions. McManus et al (2004) suggested that:

> '...stress is not a characteristic of jobs but of doctors, different doctors in the same job being no more similar in their stress and burnout than different doctors in different jobs.'

Burnout in trainees profoundly impairs their ability to learn, as this description suggests:

> 'What started out as important, meaningful and challenging work, becomes unpleasant, unfulfilling and meaningless. Energy turns into exhaustion, involvement turns into cynicism, and efficacy turns into ineffectiveness.' (Maslach et al, 2001)

McKimm (2009) notes the importance of being sensitive to the support needs arising during periods of change and transition, and allowing a period of free 'talk time' at the end of regular supervision meetings.

The value of mentoring

> 'The role of the mentor is vital for those in and out of training schemes. Good mentors are extraordinary people: they have the ability to turn around failing careers and change failure into success.' (Lake, 2009)

Ensuring that trainees feel supported in the workplace is a key to the progression of trainees in difficulty. Mentoring was highlighted in a report by the Standing Committee on Postgraduate Medical and Dental Education (1998) as a valuable framework for personal, professional and educational support. It describes mentoring as fundamentally a voluntary relationship, which should be:

> '...positive, facilitative, and developmental...not related to, nor...part of organisational systems of assessment or monitoring of performance.' (Standing Committee on Postgraduate Medical and Dental Education, 1998)

Fraser (2004) describes mentorship as a relationship akin to that in the apprenticeship model, characterized by its breadth of compass – it is more than a relationship between a junior and an educational supervisor, which may only last 6 months – it may span a much longer period of time – perhaps years – from early postgraduate days to positions of seniority. A mentoring relationship with a direct clinical supervisor may not be possible. This is partly because of the brevity of contact, but more fundamentally, because the employee–employer relationship may incorporate dynamics that run counter to the essence of the mentoring relationship.

A trainee's formally designated educational supervisor may maintain contact with his/her mentee for a longer period of time, and be a little more remote from the work pressures than the direct clinical supervisor, thus fulfilling some of the preferred benefits of a mentor.

The Standing Committee on Postgraduate Medical and Dental Education recommends that informal mentoring structures be encouraged. Fraser (2004) agrees: the ideal relationship of mentor and mentee happens unusually, is informal, and usually as a result of deliberate choice by the junior of one more senior from whom they are ready to seek counsel. Whether this kind of relationship can be organized by an external agency is debatable, but Fraser suggests that at least, senior doctors should be asked to volunteer as mentors – to fill the role of 'teaching, coaching, supporting, counselling, and sharing information with the protégé.'

Conclusions

It is important to recognize and respond to potential 'early warning signs' that may suggest difficulties in training. Careful diagnosis can lead to appropriate management planning with the rest of the team.

KEY POINTS

- Seek to create an open, trusting relationship with all trainees where the interplay between work and life is acknowledged and respected. Do not underestimate the power of regular 'developmental conversations' with all trainees.

- Know the local educational and human resources structures and use them well. A trainee in difficulty is likely to require advice and guidance from a range of people, as will the supervisor. Remember that trainees in difficulty are also employees in difficulty who may put patient care or safety at risk. Involve appropriate colleagues with specialist skills within the organization and local deanery at an early stage.

- Keep contemporaneous records of all encounters with the trainee, in accordance with employer, deanery and professional body guidelines.

- Use workplace-based assessments diagnostically. Be explicit about causes for concern and set realistic goals for improvement which are monitored.

References

Firth-Cozens J (2003) Doctors, their wellbeing and their stress. *BMJ* **326**: 670–1

Fraser A (2004) Mentoring resident doctors. *N Z Med J* **117**(1204) www.nzma.org.nz/journal/117-1204/1124/content.pdf (accessed 16 April 2010)

General Medical Council (2006) *Good Medical Practice*. General Medical Council, London (www.gmc-uk.org/guidance/good_medical_practice/duties_of_a_doctor.asp accessed 21 April 2010)

Lake J (2009) Doctors in difficulty and revalidation: where next for the medical profession? *Med Educ* **43**(7): 611–12

Launer J (2006) Supervision, mentoring and coaching: one-to-one learning encounters in medical education. Association for the Study of Medical Education, Edinburgh

Maslach C, Schaufeli W, Leiter M (2001) Job burnout. *Annu Rev Psychol* **52**: 397–422

Maslow A (1943) A theory for human motivation. *Psychol Rev* **50**(4): 370–96

McKimm J (2009) Personal support and mentoring. In: Cooper N, Forrest K, eds. *Essential Guide to Educational Supervision in Postgraduate Medical Education*. Wiley-Blackwell, BMJ Books, London: 12–28

McManus I, Keeling A, Paice E (2004) Stress, burnout and doctors' attitudes to work are determined by personality and learning style. A twelve year longitudinal study of UK medical graduates. *BMC Medicine* **2**: 29 www.biomedcentral.com/1741-7015/2/29 (accessed 7 September 2009)

Moore S, Kuol N (2007) Matters of the heart: Exploring the emotional dimensions of educational experience in recollected accounts of excellent teaching. *International Journal for Academic Development* *12*(2): 87–98

National Association of Clinical Tutors (2008) Managing trainees in difficulty: Practical advice for educational and clinical supervisors. www.nact.org.uk/pdf_documents/nactdocs/Trainees%20in%20Difficulty%20Jan%2008.pdf (accessed 7 September 2009)

Paice E (2006) The role of education and training. In: Cox J, King J, Hutchinson A, McAvoy P, eds. *Understanding Doctors Performance*. Radcliffe, Oxford: 78–90

Standing Committee on Postgraduate Medical and Dental Education (1998) *Supporting doctors and dentists at work: an inquiry into mentoring*. SCOPME, Department of Health, London

Swanwick T (2005) Informal learning in postgraduate medical education: from cognitivism to culturism. *Med Educ* **39**: 859–65

Turnbull S (2000) The role of emotion in situated learning and communities of practice. The role of emotion in situated learning and communities of practice. In: *Proceedings of the Conference on Working Knowledge, 10–13 December 2000, Sydney*. National Centre for Vocational Education Research, Adelaide, Australia: 453–62

Diversity, equal opportunities and human rights

Judy McKimm and Helen Webb

Equality and diversity are central to education and health services, in terms of both employment and service delivery. Clinical teachers need to be able to support students and trainees around equality issues, have the confidence to challenge discriminatory practice and provide an inclusive and safe learning and teaching environment.

This chapter provides an introduction to equality and diversity, discrimination and social identity in relation to medical and health professions' education. It provides an overview of relevant legal frameworks, considers ways of challenging discrimination and discusses how equality principles can be applied to the education and training of health professionals.

Equality and diversity

Although sometimes used interchangeably, the terms 'equality' and 'diversity' are not the same. Equality is about 'creating a fairer society, where everyone can participate and has the opportunity to fulfil their potential' (Department of Health, 2004). It is about identifying patterns of experience based on group identity, and the challenging processes that limit individuals' 'potential' health and life chances.

One example is occupational segregation. Women make up almost 75% of the NHS workforce but are concentrated in the lower-paid occupational areas: nursing, allied health professionals, administrative workers and ancillary workers (Department of Health, 2005). People from black and minority ethnic groups comprise 39.1% of hospital medical staff yet they comprise only 22.1% of all hospital medical consultants (Department of Health, 2005).

An equalities approach understands that social identity – in terms of gender, race or ethnicity, disability, age, social class, sexuality and religion or faith – impacts on life experiences (*Table 20.1*).

Table 20.1. Social identity – key terms	
Class	Class refers to hierarchical differences between individuals or groups in societies or cultures. Factors that determine class may vary widely from one society to another. However, economic disadvantage and barriers to access services are major issues within class discrimination
Disability	The definition of disability in the Disability Discrimination Act 1995 covers anyone with an impairment which has a substantial and long-term (at least 12 months) effect on their ability to carry out day-to-day activities such as mobility, speech, hearing or eyesight, memory or ability to concentrate, learning or understanding, or continence. The definition includes long-term illnesses such as human immunodeficiency virus infection, cancer and multiple sclerosis, from the point of diagnosis
Racial groups	A racial group is a group of people defined by their race, colour, nationality (including citizenship), ethnicity or national origins
Sexuality	This term refers to the general preference of people. It is an alternative term for 'sexual orientation' and is the term currently used

Diversity literally means difference. When it is used as a contrast or addition to equality, it is about recognizing individual as well as group differences, treating people as individuals, and placing positive value on diversity. Individual and group diversity needs to be considered in order to ensure that everybody's needs and requirements are understood and responded to within employment practice and service design and delivery.

A commitment to equality in addition to recognition of diversity means that different can be equal.

Why are equality and diversity important?

Equality and diversity are becoming more important in all aspects of our lives:

- We live in an increasingly diverse society and need to be able to respond appropriately and sensitively to this diversity. Learners in the health-care setting will reflect this diversity
- Organizations emphasize that successful implementation of equality and diversity in all aspects of work ensures that colleagues, staff and students are valued, motivated and treated fairly
- We must ensure we avoid discrimination, working within the equality and human rights legal framework covering employment practices and service delivery.

Understanding how discrimination can impact on individuals' lives is essential to prevent potential discrimination in teaching and learning situations to ensure confidence in dealing with discrimination issues if and when they arise. It is important that we also identify the links between social identities and individuality and/or a state and situation. Bad treatment can be multi-layered and occur because of an aspect of individuality, e.g. some aspect of personal appearance, size or personal likes, or someone's state or situation, e.g. homelessness, being a lone parent, misuse of drugs or alcohol, citizen status or health.

Valuing diversity

An individual learner's social identity may impact on his/her experience of a programme, teaching session or clinical activity. Discrimination works in practice through stereotyping, making assumptions, patronizing, humiliating and disrespecting people or taking some people less seriously.

The following principles help to ensure that we value diversity and consider the individual's social identity appropriately in clinical teaching. We must:

- Recognize that we need to respect learners as individuals and respond to them and their social identity in an individual manner
- Understand that treating people fairly does not mean treating people in the same way – we need to recognize difference and respond appropriately
- Try to increase our knowledge and understanding of aspects of social identity that may be different from our own
- Avoid stereotyping or making assumptions about learners based on their social identity
- Recognize that some course content may impact on some learners in a negative or difficult way
- Recognize that the course structure, e.g. timing of lectures, unsociable hours, weekend working, may impact on some learners more than others
- Recognize that your own social identity may impact on learners in different ways
- Avoid using inappropriate and disrespectful language relating to social identity (Lewis and Habershaw, 1990).

Cultural competence

Organizations are increasingly recognizing that cultural competence (linked to cultural sensitivity, cultural awareness, cultural knowledge or valuing of different cultures) is important. Cultural competence can be defined as 'a set of congruent behaviours, attitudes, and policies that come together in a system, agency, or among professionals that enables effective work in cross-cultural situations' (Cross et al, 1989). Cultural competence recognizes that the diversity of employees and service users can be challenging with barriers around, for example, language, cultural misunderstandings and interpretation. These challenges need to be effectively addressed at all levels of organizations and within education and service delivery.

Institutional discrimination

Institutional discrimination refers to discrimination that has been incorporated into the structures, processes and procedures of organizations, either because of prejudice or because of failure to take into account the particular needs of different social identities.

Three features distinguish institutional discrimination from other random individual forms of bad treatment:

1. It is triggered by social identity: the discrimination impacts on groups (or individuals because they are members of that group)
2. It is systematic and built into:
   - Laws, rules and regulations, e.g. selection criteria for jobs or courses, laws such as the minimum wage, pension regularities
   - 'The way we do things round here', including the use of authority and discretion, e.g. how training opportunities are allocated, how flexibility in learning practices is authorized
   - The popular culture and ways of describing 'normality', e.g. long working hours culture or expectations.
3. It results in patterns. Incidents of discrimination may appear isolated or random but where institutional discrimination occurs they are part of a wider, often hidden, pattern of events. Patterns of discrimination can often be surfaced by effective organizational information relating to social identity. For example, which groups of people:
   - Get promoted in an organization?
   - Get accepted onto a training course?
   - Leave an organization after 6 months of employment?

The answers to these questions (obtained through systematic monitoring) may indicate that some people experience the organization in a different or more negative way than others.

The legal context

As a clinical teacher, understanding the legal framework regarding equality helps you to relate this framework to your everyday role. The UK framework comprises two elements:

- The anti-discriminatory framework (which gives individuals a route to raise complaints of discrimination around employment and service delivery)
- The public duties (which place a proactive duty on organizations to address institutional discrimination).

Overview of anti-discriminatory framework

The main pieces of legislation that support the equality and diversity agenda are the Sex Discrimination Act 1975, the Race Relations Act 1976, the Disability Discrimination Act 1995, the Employment Equality (Sexual Orientation) and (Religious Belief) Regulations 2003, the Employment Equality (Age) Regulations 2006 and the Equality Act 2006 (covers service delivery in relation to sexual orientation and religious belief) (*Table 20.2*).

The Special Educational Needs (SEN) and Disability Act 2001 extended the Disability Discrimination Act 1995 to education with effect from September 2002. This act requires teachers to explore the provision of reasonable adjustments for students who may have disabilities, including learning disabilities, to enable them to participate effectively.

In April 2010, a new Equality Act passed through the House of Commons which seeks to harmonise existing legislation and extend it to

Table 20.2. Who is protected?	
Gender	Women, men, people in relation to gender reassignment
Race/ethnicity	Anyone in relation to ethnic origin, nationality, colour or culture
Disability	Anyone with an impairment that has a substantial and long-term effect on his/her ability to carry out day-to-day activities
Sexuality	Lesbians, gay men, bisexual and heterosexual people
Religion/belief	Anyone in relation to religious or philosophical belief, including not having a particular religion or belief
Age	Anyone of any age

cover age, disability, sex, gender reassignment, sexual orientation, race, religion or belief and, in many but not all instances, marriage and civil partnerships. The Act will be implemented throughout 2010/11, and the final details of the Act are still potentially subject to change. Key points of the law include:

- Introducing a new public sector duty to consider reducing socio-economic inequalities
- Introducing an Equality Duty on public bodies
- Banning age discrimination outside the workplace
- Requiring greater openness from public bodies on gender pay and employment equality reporting
- Extending the scope to use positive action
- Protecting carers from discrimination
- Strengthening protection from discrimination for disabled people
- Protecting people from dual discrimination – direct discrimination because of a combination of two protected characteristics.

Key legal principles

The legal framework gives rise to key principles (*Table 20.3*):

- Direct discrimination
- Indirect discrimination
- Harassment
- Reasonable adjustment
- Positive action
- Genuine occupational qualification
- Victimization.

Public duties

In 2000, the first public duty covering race was introduced, followed in 2006 and 2007 by duties covering disability and gender respectively. Under the Equality Act 2010 the duties have been extended to cover all equality strands. In addition a new socio-economic duty has been suggested. The equality duty will be introduced in 2011. Until this time, organizations should continue to meet their obligations under the race, disability and gender duties. The duties apply to all public bodies, including local authorities, education, police forces, national health services, NHS trusts and bodies. It is through the implementation of these public duties that organizations will identify and address institutional discrimination. Each public duty requires

Table 20.3. Equality and diversity – key terms

Discrimination	Discrimination is less favourable or bad treatment of someone because of one or more aspects of their social identity. Direct discrimination is less favourable treatment on the grounds of someone's social identity which results in an adverse impact and cannot be justified. Indirect discrimination is when a rule, condition or requirement is applied to everyone but some people find this more difficult to fulfil, causing an adverse impact which cannot be justified.
Genuine qualification	If an employer requires a person of a specific social identity for personal services or occupational 'authenticity', they can request a Genuine Occupational Qualification or a Genuine Qualification Occupational Requirement from the Equal Opportunities Commission.
Harassment	Harassment occurs if A's conduct has the purpose or effect of violating B's dignity or of creating an offensive environment – one that is intimidating, hostile, degrading or humiliating.
Positive action	In the areas of training, recruitment, and membership of organizations such as trade unions, if a gender or racial group has been under-represented in the previous 12 months, employers can offer selective training programmes, advertise to encourage applications or train staff responsible for selection. This is positive action. Offering someone a job or promotion on the basis of their gender, race etc is positive discrimination which was illegal in the past. However, the Equality Act 2010 states that in certain circumstances, organizations be allowed to recruit and promote in favour of under-represented groups. Quotas (as opposed to targets) are illegal.
Prejudice	Prejudice ('prejudging') describes the feelings that individuals have about other individuals or groups, feelings that are often unfounded and based on stereotypes. We all have prejudices based on our own experiences and indirect experience, e.g. through the mass media, but usually learn to overcome these feelings, or at least control how we behave with others and what we say. Discrimination can be seen as 'prejudice put into practice', where people let their prejudices affect what they say about and how they behave towards others.
Reasonable adjustment	Reasonable adjustments are steps which an employer or service provider may have to take in relation to a disabled person in order to comply with the Act, e.g. making adjustments to premises, allocating some of the disabled person's duties to another person, altering their working hours, allowing them to be absent during working hours for rehabilitation, assessment or treatment, acquiring or modifying equipment, modifying instructions or reference manuals or procedures for testing or assessment, providing a reader or interpreter.
Victimisation	Victimisation arises where a person treats another less favourably because that person has asserted their rights under the Equality Act 2010 if, for example, that person has brought proceedings, or given evidence or information in connection with proceedings, under the Act.

organizations to:

- Produce a race, disability and gender equality scheme
- Carry out impact assessments on their functions, policies and practices
- Carry out equalities monitoring and take action to redress any imbalance
- Publish the results of any work undertaken.

A summary of current public duties is provided in *Table 20.4*.

Human rights

Human rights are the basic rights and principles that belong to every person in the world. They are based on the core principles of fairness, respect, equality, dignity and autonomy. Human rights protect an individual's freedom to control his/her day-to-day life and effectively participate in all aspects of public life in a fair and equal way.

Human rights help individuals to flourish and achieve potential through:

- Being safe and protected from harm
- Being treated fairly and with dignity
- Being able to live the life you choose
- Taking an active part in your community and wider society (Equality and Human Rights Commission, 2010).

Intrinsic to these statements should be the principles of equality and diversity.

Since 1998 the UK has also included human rights within its legal framework. The Human Rights Act applies to all public authorities and

Table 20.4. Public duties and discrimination	
Race	Promote equality of opportunity
	Eliminate unlawful discrimination
	Promote good relations between different racial groups
Disability	Promote equality of opportunity
	Promote positive attitudes towards disabled people and encourage their participation in public life
	Take account of disabled people's impairments, even when this involves treating a disabled person more favourably than others
Gender	Promote equality of opportunity
	Ensure that they do not discriminate unlawfully between women and men when carrying out their employment and service functions

bodies performing a public function, and places the responsibility on all organizations to promote and protect individuals' human rights (this means treating people fairly, with dignity and respect while safeguarding the rights of the wider community) and to apply the core human rights values, of fairness, respect, equality, dignity and autonomy, to all organizational service planning and decision making.

The Human Rights Act provides a complementary legal framework to the anti-discriminatory framework and public duties. The Equality and Human Rights Commission website (www.equalityhumanrights.com) contains useful resources and information.

The learning and teaching context

As a clinical teacher you will need to role model cultural competence which may require you to challenge learners over their behaviour because you feel it is potentially discriminatory and in order to:

- Ensure you create a learning environment that is inclusive, free of discrimination and that values difference
- Reinforce the policies and procedures of your organization
- Ensure you do not breach the equalities legal framework.

Knowing what to challenge, and when to challenge, can be tricky and open to personal interpretation. There are some non-negotiables regarding inappropriate language or behaviour, e.g. swearing, language that is racist, sexist or homophobic. Questions such as 'what constitutes inappropriate banter?' or 'they meant no offence by a comment – do I still need to challenge?' are more difficult to answer.

Not challenging is not a neutral act – it can be seen as colluding behaviour and can in itself be seen as a form of discrimination.

Case scenarios

Here are some examples of remarks and situations that might be discriminatory or require challenging:

1. You observe a student talking to a patient with learning disabilities. The patient has a speech impairment which means that his speech is slow. The student continually interrupts him and finishes his sentences for him.
2. You have noticed that a trainee tends to make a number of assumptions when referring to patients' social identity. For example she often says things like 'Asian people do this' or 'gay men are known for doing that'. You are worried it may demonstrate underlying issues.

Other issues might require specific support from teachers or supervisors, for example:

3. A trainee tells you that he does not want to deal with a particular patient because he feels she is treating him in a racist manner. Can he refuse to deal with a patient on these grounds?

4. A student was diagnosed with depression 1 year ago but did not tell you until 3 months ago, when she confided in you about what she was experiencing and the treatment she was getting from her GP and therapist. A month ago she was signed off on sick leave. She returned to work last week but feels overwhelmed. She is determined to carry on with her training. What support can you provide?

Challenging behaviours: guiding principles

If in doubt about whether you should challenge someone's behaviour or not, consider the following:

- Is the banter, joke or comment excluding anyone or aimed at anyone in order to ridicule him/her?
- Could someone be offended by the behaviour?
- Is the banter, joke or behaviour open to misinterpretation or misunderstanding?
- Lack of intention is not an excuse for behaviour. You are required to consider and manage the effect of behaviour.

There is no definite way to challenge inappropriate behaviour and everyone finds their own approach to challenging effectively. The following may be useful:

- Do not punish or blame – say what is better
- Understand your audience. Think about your role in the situation – clinician, supervisor, teacher, peer, colleague, manager – and consider this in your approach
- State your position: 'That's disrespectful; we don't talk about patients like that'
- Understand the situation. Do you challenge there and then, or quietly at a later date? What will be most effective for the person involved and/or for those witnessing the incident?

Conclusions

Understanding the principles of equality and diversity and the underpinning legislative framework helps to inform teaching and learning practice and provide a more effective and inclusive learning environment. Teachers have a responsibility to challenge discriminatory practices and to use the legislation and diversity agenda to positively advocate for more equitable teaching and learning practices. This may involve:

- Ensuring that there are policies in place to deal with complaints about discrimination on any grounds
- Discussing equalities with student or trainee representatives
- Ensuring that learners know where to go if they have concerns about discrimination
- Ensuring that adequate procedures are in place for assessing and managing the needs of learners with disabilities
- Dealing properly with complaints and maintaining proper records (what may seem to be a small incident once may be part of a pattern)
- Ensuring that issues are discussed as openly as possible within an institution, while dealing with specific incidents confidentially
- Giving people feedback if they are complained about. They may be doing something that can easily be changed.

References

KEY POINTS

- Teachers have a responsibility to promote equality, recognize diversity and provide an inclusive learning environment for students and trainees.
- Many aspects of social identity impact on the learning process, both positively and negatively.
- Equality and diversity issues may arise in formal and informal learning events, in practice settings and throughout organizational systems and structures.
- Discrimination needs to be challenged, this takes both interpersonal skills and knowledge of legislation and equality principles.
- Understanding the anti-discriminatory and human rights frameworks can help teachers provide appropriate support for learners.

Cross T, Bazron B, Dennis K, Isaacs M (1989) *Towards a Culturally Competent System of Care, Volume I*. Georgetown University Child Development Center, CASSP Technical, Washington, DC

Department of Health (2004) *Sharing the Challenge, Sharing the Benefits – equality and diversity in the medical workforce directorate*. Department of Health, London

Department of Health (2005) *Promoting Equality and Human rights in the NHS: a guide for non-executive directors of boards*. Department of Health, London

Equality and Human Rights Commission (2010) Human Rights. www.equalityhumanrights. com/human-rights (accessed 23 June 2010)

Lewis V, Habeshaw S (1990) *53 Interesting Ways to Promote Equal Opportunities in Education*. Technical and Educational Services, Bristol

CHAPTER 21

Introduction to educational research

Clare Morris and Judy McKimm

Clinical teachers need to be able to make informed judgements about the quality of published educational research before drawing upon it to enhance their teaching and learning. Those wishing to conduct educational research may have to re-think the nature of 'evidence' to develop and use appropriate research approaches.

This chapter introduces some of the key debates in medical education research. It provides an overview of some of the key research methods aligned to educational research within a social science (rather than a natural science) paradigm and supports this with some examples from the literature. Common frameworks used to judge the quality and fitness for purpose of educational research are considered. Finally, some key questions to guide educational research design and implementation are suggested.

The nature of 'evidence' in educational research

> *'My own research in schools and hospitals indicated that both education and medicine are profoundly people-centred professions. Neither believes that helping people is merely a matter of a simple technical application but rather a highly skilled process in which a sophisticated judgement matches a professional decision to the unique needs of each client. Yet the two professions see the role of scientific knowledge in informing professional practice in very different ways. The kind of science, and so the kind of research, involved in each profession is very different.'* (Hargreaves, 1996).

Hargreaves' lecture provoked some very public debate about the traditions of research in medicine and education and the different understandings about the nature of 'evidence' in each (Hargreaves, 1996; Hammersley,

1997). Many commentators have noted the ways in which particular types of knowledge are elevated to hold particular status (Boaz and Ashby, 2003; Long et al, 2006) and debates about the relative value of different types of research are widespread. The details of these debates are beyond the scope of this chapter, but they highlight an important starting point. Our prior histories of research and the views we hold about learning are likely to lead us to value certain types of research above others and lead us to attempt to undertake research in particular ways. There is a risk that we are pulled into binary debates, aligning ourselves to one particular paradigm (natural science *vs* social science), research tradition (quantitative *vs* qualitative) or standpoint on learning (acquisition *vs* participation). This polarization and 'world view' may lead to methods and approaches being taken that are inappropriate for the topic or context being studied.

As Teunissen (2010) recently warned:

'when your grasp of theoretical perspectives is limited, your education and research designs are in danger of lacking profundity.'

Teunissen, like others, is critical of the atheoretical nature of much medical education research, and suggests that once a research topic has been identified, researchers then need to identify the theoretical concepts that can inform the design of the study or guide the analysis of the data (Teunissen, 2010). Others argue that part of this process involves making the conceptions of learning that underpin our approaches to educational research and practice explicit, both to ourselves (as researchers) and to others (Swanwick and Morris, 2010).

To illustrate, let us imagine we have two research teams who have been asked to conduct research into teaching and learning on ward rounds. Team one have developed expertise in research of the positivist traditions of science; they believe in the power of logic and mathematics to demonstrate 'truth' or 'proof'. They value quantitative methodologies that allow them to explore causations, correlations and significance. Their study design looks at the types of interactions between trainers and trainees on the ward round, seeking to quantify the amount of trainer and trainee talk and the number of 'teaching' *vs* 'business' types of exchanges. They decide to investigate how much 'learning' happens and, guided by what Sfard (1998) calls the 'acquisition metaphor', seek to capture the amount of knowledge acquired by doing some before and after measures using a multiple choice questionnaire assessment. They observe and record interactions (number of different type, mean length of utterance) during consultations and seek to find statistical significances between different types of rounds.

Team two, on the other hand, are trained in the social science tradition and value qualitative methodologies that allow them to shed light on behaviours, opinions, experiences and feelings. They decide to explore different stakeholder perspectives on the value of ward rounds for learning purposes, interviewing trainers, trainees and other members of the multidisciplinary team. They too want to look at the ways in which 'learning' is fostered by ward rounds and, guided by what Sfard (1998) calls the 'participation metaphor', they observe ward rounds with a view to revealing the ways in which trainees are 'socialised' into certain ways of thinking about and talking about patients. They also look at the extent to which trainees are provided with the types of learning opportunities that enable them to become full participants in the ward round, eventually leading rounds themselves. They use interview and observational methods, drawing on the traditions of ethnography. Each research team has designed studies that have the potential to inform the ways in which trainee learning can best be supported on ward rounds. The main contrasts between the ways in which they approach their research lie in the ways in which they conceptualize the world, the types of questions they ask and try to answer, and the methods they adopt to try and answer those questions.

Table 21.1 brings these hypothetical issues to life, by drawing on examples of published research about learning on ward rounds. The last example, Dornan et al (2006), has a broader remit, but is included as an example of systematic reviews in medical education. Column one summarizes the authors' aims and purposes, column two aims to turn these into the types of questions that appear to underpin the studies and column three illustrates the different approaches adopted.

Fitness for purpose in educational research

All clinical teachers are likely to engage with educational research as consumers if not producers. Davies (1999) suggests that in order to make use of existing research evidence and judge fitness for purpose in relation to their own work, all those involved in education should be able to pose answerable questions about education and to retrieve and adopt a critical stance to existing evidence. The 'Best Evidence Medical Education' movement is based on a similar philosophy, with advocates arguing that:

'...being a competent education practitioner in both the clinic and the classroom includes being able to understand and integrate evidence of effectiveness, with theory and experience, into teaching practice' (Hammick and Haig, 2007).

A sensible starting point for all educational research might be to ask 'what do we know works' and, equally importantly, 'what do we know doesn't work?' Judging the quality and fitness for purpose of existing research is an important prerequisite for all medical education researchers, who need to

Table 21.1. Studies of learning on ward rounds

Study: stated aims and purposes	Assumed underpinning research question(s)	Methodology and methods
Patterns of interaction among team members, learners' perceptions of the educational utility of rounds (Walton and Steinert, 2010)	What is the nature, frequency and duration of interactions between trainers and trainees on rounds? What are the perceived educational purposes of rounds?	Direct observation of rounds, with simultaneous data-coding (type and duration of interaction) Completion of Likert-scale questionnaire, to signify level of agreement with statements
To explore the teaching and learning processes that occur during rounds and the implications for their role in medical education (Kuper et al, 2010)	What happens during ward rounds and how might we understand this? To what extent do trainers and trainees share similar views on the educational value of rounds?	Ethnography: non-participant observation Semi-structured interviews with trainers and trainees
To explore staff, patient and parent views on paediatric ward rounds and to use outcomes to inform changes to approach (Birtwistle et al, 2000)	What are doctors', nurses', patients' and parents' attitudes towards ward rounds? How might this inform the development of our approach to ward rounds?	Unstructured interviews with each group (doctors and nurses, patients and parents) to determine key themes for a Likert-scale questionnaire administered to a larger population

Table 21.1. Studies of learning on ward rounds (cont)

Study: stated aims and purposes	Assumed underpinning research question(s)	Methodology and methods
To identify ways to maximize educational opportunities on ward rounds as part of a widerproject to improve on-the-job learning (Stanley, 1998)	To what extent are ward rounds currently structured and conducted in ways that promote junior doctor learning? How might learning opportunities be enhanced?	Observation of ward rounds, with notes taken on structure, routines and trainer-trainee contribution Classification of types of rounds and critique of educational value
To identify final year medical students' deficiencies in conducting rounds in order to develop appropriate teaching and assessment tools for learning (Nikendei et al, 2008)	How prepared are medica students to conduct ward rounds? What are the types of difficulties medical students encounter when conducting a ward round?	Observation and analysis of simulated ward rounds with medical student volunteers
To establish the validity of a task-specific checklist designed to guide and evaluate trainee performance when conducting ward rounds (Norgaard et al, 2004)	How confident can we be in the content and construct validity of the ward round checklist?	Content validity assessed by a Likert-based questionnaire, construct validity assessed by piloting the tool while observing doctors of different levels of seniority conduct a round
To identify the effects of early clinical exposure in medical education (Dornan et al, 2006)	How can experience in clinical and community settings contribute to early medical education?	Systematic review of existing literatures

avoid the trap of using frameworks from one tradition to judge the quality of research in another tradition. A number of frameworks exist that seek to counter this risk. One example (*Figure 21.1*) focuses on quality:

'The traditional approach to quality assessment has been to focus on methodological rigour. We have discussed a broader definition of quality that pays closer attention to the ways in which the research will be used and the ways in which it is presented. We have identified a number of dimensions of quality that seem to apply to a variety of types of research. Each of these represents an important dimension of quality assessment' (Boaz and Ashby, 2003).

A further helpful model is the 'TAPUPAS' model (Pawson et al, 2003), arising from a knowledge review conducted for the Social Care Institute for Excellence which is designed to judge the quality of all types of knowledge, including that generated by research:

- Transparency – are the reasons for it clear?
- Accuracy – is it honestly based on relevant evidence?
- Purposivity – is the method used suitable for the aims of the work?
- Utility – does it provide answers to the questions it sets?
- Propriety – is it legal and ethical?
- Accessibility – can you understand it?
- Specificity – does it meet the quality standards already used for this type of knowledge?

These two models can be used to guide a critique of existing research, or help researchers plan research of high quality.

Figure 21.1. Dimensions of research quality.
Adapted from Boaz and Ashby (2003).

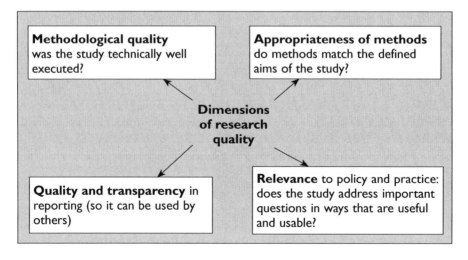

Designing educational research

So far we have looked at the ways in which different research traditions position researchers to ask particular types of questions and adopt particular types of research approaches. We have also noted the importance of adopting a critical stance to all types of 'evidence', including that in published research. Kuper et al (2008a) suggest that readers of qualitative studies should ask six key questions:

1. Was the sample used in the study appropriate to the research question?
2. Were the data collected appropriately?
3. Were the data analysed appropriately?
4. Can the results of this study be transferred to my own setting?
5. Does the study adequately address potential ethical issues, including reflexivity (position of researcher)?
6. Overall, is what the researchers did clear?

These questions can also be used to guide study design. This section provides a brief overview of key issues in designing educational research in the qualitative tradition. This starts from identifying appropriate research questions and concludes with some key points about data analysis. *Table 21.2* provides a 'quick guide' to designing and conducting a qualitative study. In reality, the stages are often overlapping with data collection and analysis being iterative and mutually informing.

Research question and design

Steps one to three are all about identifying the ways in which you will approach your research questions and research design. You should also consider how you will analyse your research data: qualitative data analysis can be very resource intensive. Qualitative research is described as:

Table 21.2. Seven steps to designing a qualitative study

1. Identify starting position, including theoretical position and what previous studies say about the topic
2. Identify your research questons
3. Decide upon research methods
4. Identify an appropriate sampling strategy
5. Identify ethical issues: gain appropriate permissions
6. Gain access to the field and gather data
7. Analyse data and interpret findings (triangulate where possible and refer back to the published literature)

> '...any type of research that produces findings not arrived at by statistical procedures or other means of quantification. It can refer to research about persons' lives, lived experiences, behaviours, emotions and feelings as well as about organizational functioning, social movements, cultural phenomena and interactions between nations.' (Strauss and Corbin, 1998)

Qualitative research often adopts what is described as a 'grounded theory' approach, where the theories emerge from the data (from the ground up) in an iterative fashion. This contrasts with defining a hypothesis and then designing a study to seek data to prove or disprove the thesis which uses identified conceptual or theoretical tools analytically. For those used to working in the natural sciences or experimental research, the former approach and the 'evidence' that emerges from it can appear 'fuzzy' and 'soft'. However, both approaches are equally valid but draw from and seek to explain different phenomena. Kuper et al (2008b) suggest that quantitative research focuses on answering the questions 'what?', 'how much?' and 'why?' whereas qualitative research focuses on answering the questions 'why?' and 'how?'. Increasingly, researchers are using mixed methods drawn from both qualitative and quantitative approaches, but any methods chosen need to be appropriate to the topic and context of the study.

So, a grounded approach might ask a more open question such as 'how do medical students experience learning in the workplace?', whereas a theoretically driven approach might ask 'to what extent can medical students experiences of learning in the workplace be described as time spent in Communities of Practice? (as defined by Lave and Wenger, 1991)'. The research question then leads to the identification of appropriate research methods. The first question might lead us to interview medical students, at different stages in training, individually or in groups. The second question may also lead us to use interview methods, with the questions shaped by core tenets of the theories we are drawing upon (for example, opportunities for legitimate peripheral participation). We may also wish to use some observational methods to triangulate these accounts with what we actually observe in the workplace. *Table 21.3* describes common educational research methods.

Sampling methods

Steps four and five are also important preparatory stages. Sampling methods used in qualitative studies are described as theoretical or purposeful, with the emphasis being not on gaining a 'representative' sample, as is the tradition in the scientific paradigm, but on gaining a sample that is 'representative of the

Table 21.3. Common educational research methods

Method	Description
Action research	'a method that involves the researcher in working in collaboration with participants through cycles of evaluation and development to produce positive changes to practice or relationships' (Kuper et al, 2008b)
Systematic review	'review of a clearly formulated question that uses systematic and explicit methods to identify, select and critically appraise relevant research and to collect and analyse data from the studies that are included in the review. Statistical methods (meta-analysis) may or may not be used to analyse and summarise the results of the included studies' (Clark and Oxman, 2003)
Case study	A case study is an in-depth, detailed, systematic contextual analysis and exploration of a group, organization, event or individual, usu ally carried out over time. This form of research uses a range of methods, seeks multiple sources of evidence and often generates hypotheses or ideas for further, wider exploration or study.
Ethnography	Traditional participant observation is now questioned on ethical grounds (as the researcher status is hidden from the community being observed). Non-participant observation, however, means you seek to gain trust and cooperation, with your observer status agreed by the group. This allows the researcher to observe activi ties and to engage with group members, to discuss what has been seen and seek further information or explanation.
Interview	Interviews are usually carried out on a one-to-one basis, face to face or by telephone or other communication media. They are typi cally structured (with a list of questions about the topic from which the interviewer does not deviate) or semi structured (with a framework, but allowing for probing into areas or following ideas).
Focus groups	This is a small group meeting or interview, comprising members of a wider community, who are sampled through facilitated open dis cussion on a specific topic to elicit their opinions or feelings. Like interviews, focus group meetings can be very loosely or tightly structured.

population being studied', seeking to involve those who are most and least representative as well as the 'typical'. Ethical considerations are particularly important in educational research which is often 'insider' research, where you may already have a pre-existing relationship with those you are studying (as colleague, teacher or manager). Issues of power and authority are explicitly considered in qualitative research, along with reflexivity: the position and impact of the researcher on the research process and those they are researching. The British Educational Research Association

(2004) provides comprehensive guidance on these issues. The National Research Ethics Service also provides helpful guidance on the types of study that require ethical approval, distinguishing between research, audit and evaluation studies. Having gained appropriate permissions, the next stage is to gain 'access to the field', where issues of consent are vitally important. It is important to avoid any actions that imply coercion, with participants being able to opt in and opt out of the study at any point.

Gathering and analysing data

Steps six and seven are separated out in the guide, but in reality are often closely connected. During this stage you may begin to undertake some preliminary analysis, which feeds into subsequent data collection as you seek to gain a 'rich picture' of the issues you are exploring. Qualitative researchers often talk about reaching a point of 'data saturation' where new data collected fails to yield any new or significant insights into the issue being explored. In adopting a grounded approach, it is likely that data analysis will be based upon a first coding of data (into content categories) and thematic analysis, which seeks to make connections between ideas and to shed light on new or emerging phenomenon or understandings. A theoretically-driven approach will typically ask particular questions of the data. A detailed account of data analysis methods is outside the scope of this article, but it is worth noting that qualitative methods have their own rigour and that analysis is enhanced by data 'triangulation'. This may mean using multiple methods of data collection, different study samples, seeking different perspectives on the same research questions, or returning to your respondents with your analysis of data for their viewpoints.

Of course, designing and carrying out your study is only part of the activity – it is also important to think through who the audience will be for your research output and how you can best disseminate the findings. Owing to their often contextually-specific nature, qualitative studies are not 'generalizable' in the ways that quantitative studies claim to be. However, they have high explanatory power, their findings can be transferred to other contexts and they can influence policy and practice as a result. Together, the approaches have the potential to yield powerful insights into medical learning and practice.

Conclusions

High quality educational research in health and medicine provides the information and evidence needed to improve the quality of learning, teaching and assessment and ultimately to improve patient care. An appreciation that educational research draws on approaches and methods from both scientific and social science disciplines will support clinical teachers in being able to appraise the evidence that results from such studies as well as participate in research activities themselves.

KEY POINTS

- Clinical teachers should be mindful of the fact that their prior histories of research and education will influence the value placed on certain types of research and the types of questions they seek to answer.

- The main contrasts between quantitative and qualitative research lie in the ways in which they conceptualize the world, the types of questions they ask and the methods they use to try and answer those questions.

- Clinical teachers should adopt an informed and critical stance to published educational research in order to make judgements about fitness for purpose and the relevance of the study to their own areas of practice.

- A number of helpful frameworks exist to guide the critical appraisal of published research; they may also inform the design of useful and usable research.

- Well-designed educational research poses answerable questions about education, is theoretically informed and seeks alignment between purposes and methods.

References

Birtwistle L, Houghton J, Rostill H (2000) A review of a surgical ward round in a large paediatric hospital: does it achieve its aims? *Med Educ* **30:** 398–403

Boaz A, Ashby D (2003) *Fit for Purpose? Assessing research quality for evidence based policy and practice.* ESRC UK Centre for Evidence Based Policy and Practice, London

British Educational Research Association (2004) *Revised Ethical Guidelines for Educational Research.* www.bera.ac.uk/publications/guidelines/ (accessed 17 June 2010)

Clark M, Oxman AD (2003) *Cochrane Reviewers' Handbook 4.2.0.* The Cochrane Library, Oxford

Davies P (1999) What is evidence based education? *British Journal of Educational Studies* 47(2): 108–21

Dornan T, Littlewood S, Margolis SA, Scherpbier A, Spencer A, Ypinazar V (2006) How can experience in clinical and community settings contribute to early medical education? A BEME systematic review. BEME Guide No 6. *Med Teach* **28**(1): 3–18

Hargreaves DH (1996) The Teacher Training Agency Annual Lecture 1996. Teaching as a research-based profession: possibilities and prospects. http://eppi.ioe.ac.uk/cms/Portals/0/PDF%20reviews%20and%20summaries/TTA%20Hargreaves%20lecture.pdf (accessed 29 May 2010)

Hammersley M (1997) Educational Research and Teaching; a response to David Hargreaves' TTA lecture. *Br Educ Res J* **23**: 141–61

Hammick M, Haig A (2007) The Best Evidence Medical Education Collaboration: processes, products and principles. *Clin Teach* **4**: 42–45

Kuper A, Lingard L, Levinson W (2008a) Qualitative research: critically appraising qualitative research. *BMJ* **337**: 687–9

Kuper A, Reeves S, Levinson W (2008b) Qualitative research: an introduction to reading or appraising qualitative research. *BMJ* **337**: 404–7

Kuper A, Zur Nedden N, Etchells E, Shadowitz S, Reeves S (2010) Teaching and learning in morbidity and mortality rounds: an ethnographic study. *Med Educ* **44**: 559–69

Lave J, Wenger E (1991) *Situated learning. Legitimate peripheral participation.* Cambridge University Press, Cambridge

Long AF, Grayson L, Boaz A (2006) Assessing the quality of knowledge in social care: exploring the potential of a set of generic standards. *Br J Soc Work* **36**: 207–26

Nikendei C, Kraus B, Schrauth M, Briem S, Junger J (2008) Ward rounds: how prepared are future doctors? *Med Teach* **30**: 88–91

Norgaard K, Ringsted C, Dolmans D (2004) Validation of a checklist to assess ward round performance in internal medicine. *Med Educ* **38**: 700–7

Pawson R, Boaz A, Grayson L, Long AF, Barnes C (2003) Types and Quality of Knowledge in Social Care. Knowledge Review 3. Social Care Institute for Excellence (SCIE), London (www.scie.org.uk/publications/knowledgereviews/kr03.asp accessed 18 June 2010)

Sfard A (1998) On two metaphors for learning and the dangers of choosing just one. *Educational Researcher* **27**: 4–13

Stanley P (1998) Structuring ward rounds for learning: can opportunities be created? *Med Educ* **32**: 239–43

Strauss A, Corbin J (1998) *Basics of Qualitative Research. Techniques and Procedures for Developing Grounded Theory.* Sage, London

Swanwick T, Morris C (2010) Shifting conceptions of learning in the workplace. *Med Educ* **44**: 538–9

Teunissen P (2010) Commentary: On the transfer of theory to the practice of research and education. *Med Educ* **44**: 534–5

Walton J, Steinert Y (2010) Patterns of interaction during ward rounds: implications for work-based learning. *Med Educ* **44**: 550–8

CHAPTER 22

Professional development of medical educators

Tim Swanwick and Judy McKimm

Clinicians are increasingly involved in teaching, learning, assessment and supervisory activities with medical students, trainees and other health professionals. Participation in professional development pathways and activities in medical education enables clinical teachers to provide high quality education and training.

This chapter explores the role of professional development for clinical teachers in assisting individual teachers and organizations to deliver more effective and relevant education and training. It considers the needs of clinical teachers and the different opportunities, roles and activities available to medical educators.

Background and context

In 2010 we celebrate the centenary of Abraham Flexner's seminal report on the transformation of American medical school system (Flexner, 1910), a report that led to the structures of basic medical education that we see today. Flexner would not have recognized the complex structures, management and quality assurance arrangements of our postgraduate training, and the energy and resources being invested in regulatory systems to ensure the ongoing personal and professional development of practising clinicians. Medical education in the 21st century is a lifelong affair spanning three sectors: undergraduate, postgraduate and the continuing professional development of established clinicians.

Medical education's aim is to supply society with knowledgeable, skilled and up-to-date healthcare workers who undertake to maintain and develop their expertise over a lifetime career. Medicine occupies a privileged position in society and, as a result, has set itself apart from the mainstream.

However, in common with other areas of higher and professional education, three distinct trends have come to prominence in recent years: increasing accountability, a discourse of excellence and the 'professionalization' of medical educators (Swanwick, 2008).

A sense of increased accountability permeates medical education from top to bottom. The blossoming of regulatory requirements and a centralization of curricula by institutions and Royal Colleges has moved the medical teacher from a position of independence (and idiosyncracy) to a one where prescribed educational outcomes must be delivered, assessments performed to demand and student evaluations scrutinized and acted upon. Heightened levels of accountability exist not just to institutions but also to the end user, and students and trainees come with increasing expectations for high quality teaching and training. Most importantly, accountability is a key facet of a new social compact with patients; a compact, no longer based on blind and unquestioning trust, but on true partnership in which patients are key stakeholders in the education and training of the future and existing medical workforce.

In some ways the 'pursuit of excellence', has been a response to the above. Excellence (and related superlatives such as 'world-classness') is part of a discourse that pervades the public sector and is exemplified in documents such as Professor Sir John Tooke's report on the UK's reform of postgraduate training *Aspiring to Excellence* (Tooke, 2008) and Lord Darzi's wide-ranging policy for reform *A High Quality Workforce* (Darzi, 2008). It is now formally recognized that the quality of medical teaching and training is inextricably linked to the quality of patient care. And quality in medical education, increasingly informed by performance metrics and user evaluations, is very much on the health service agenda.

The final trend to highlight is that of the professionalization of medical education, a drive that comes from within medical educators themselves, a feeling of wanting 'to do it better'. Manifestations of this include an explosion of interest in professional organizations, with over 2000 delegates now regularly attending the annual conference of the Association for Medical Education in Europe, a growing number of professional associations and medical education journals, and a record number of doctors acquiring relevant postgraduate certificates, diplomas and masters degrees from an increasing number of institutions.

Frameworks for professional development

One way in which these trends are expressed is through the development of standards and frameworks for development. Standards for medical educators can be viewed as a set of Russian dolls, each set nestling inside each other but becoming more and more specific as the doll is opened. These standards reflect generic quality assurance activities and requirements from professional and statutory bodies in both undergraduate and postgraduate contexts.

All teachers in higher education, which, broadly speaking, should include the majority of medical educators, come under the UK Professional Standards Framework of the Higher Education Academy (Higher Education Academy, 2006). This overarching framework provides guidance for individual teachers and for all UK higher education institutions in creating their own staff development programmes. The Professional Standards Framework outlines key areas of activity, core knowledge and professional values against which individual teachers and programmes are accredited.

More specific still is the Professional Standards Framework of the Academy of Medical Educators launched in December 2009 (Academy of Medical Educators, 2009a). This framework is intended to 'encompass the skills, knowledge and practice required of those who perform the wide variety of educational roles undertaken within medical education' and are 'designed to assist medical educators to work towards excellence'. The six domains against which medical educators are invited to benchmark themselves, or which organizations can use as a development framework, are shown in *Figure 22.1*.

Figure 22.1. The Academy of Medical Educators (2009a) professional standards framework.

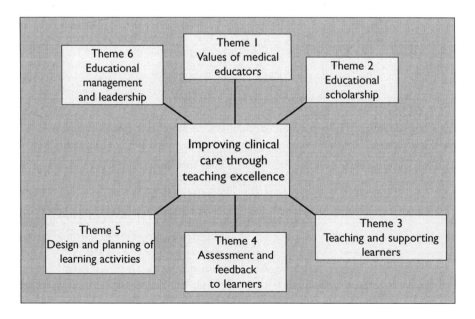

Delving further reveals sector-specific standards such as those for postgraduate supervisors produced by the Postgraduate Medical Education and Training Board (2008). Similar requirements are echoed in *Tomorrow's Doctors*, the General Medical Council's (GMC) framework of guidance for UK medical schools (GMC, 2009), which requires that all clinical teachers should participate in staff development programmes. These two regulatory organizations, Postgraduate Medical Education and Training Board and the GMC, merged into one in 2010.

Regulatory standards are further explicated in local interpretations such as the London Deanery's *Professional Development Framework for Supervisors* (London Deanery, 2009).

All of this is underpinned by professional expectations of doctors that they should be willing to teach, and if they do so, that they 'must develop the skills, attitudes and practices of a competent teacher' (GMC, 2009). All doctors with clinical teaching or training responsibilities therefore have a duty to undertake some form of educational training and development. With the imminent introduction of revalidation, implicit in the GMC's statement is that doctors who teach, train or supervise learners will need to provide evidence that they have attained the appropriate skills, attitudes and competences.

Challenges for clinical teachers

Although clinical teachers face many of the challenges that any teacher faces (such as increasing student numbers and adherence to quality assurance requirements), they carry the 'double burden' of delivering safe and high quality patient care while being responsible for teaching and training (McKimm and Swanwick, 2010).

The key challenges for clinical teachers include:
- Lack of time
- Teaching amid busy clinical workloads and service pressures
- Feelings of isolation
- Patients' rights and expectations about the quality and safety of their care that can conflict with students' or trainees' needs
- Increasing numbers of medical and other healthcare students
- Involving patients meaningfully in medical education
- Interprofessional education
- Keeping pace with new scientific and clinical knowledge
- Keeping up to date with educational requirements and advances in teaching, learning and assessment
- The impact of technology, including e-learning and simulation.

All this is in addition to the changing expectations from students and trainees and increasing demands from regulators and statutory bodies described above.

What sort of development?

Faculty development – 'teaching the teachers' or 'training the trainers' – programmes the world over have tended to focus on the improvement of individual teaching abilities across a broadly similar range of activities. A typical content list is provided in *Figure 22.2*.

Faculty development has tended to be delivered as either short courses, workshops or as accredited university awards. More innovative approaches have included longitudinal programmes – where faculty commit a proportion of their time on a regular basis over 1–2 years to develop their knowledge and skills – and the use of individual coaching, mentorship and e-learning. A systematic review looking at effectiveness of faculty development programmes (Steinert et al, 2006) found that the key features of effective development programmes were:

- Use of experiential learning
- Provision of feedback
- Effective peer/colleague relationships
- Well-designed interventions following established educational principles
- Use of a diversity of educational methods within single interventions.

Figure 22.2. Typical content of faculty development programmes.

Teaching skills and methods
Supervision
Assessment (including workplace based)
Feedback
Objective setting
Learning needs analysis
Appraisal
Careers advice
Working with portfolios
Management of poor performance
Diversity and equal opportunities
Educational theory
Small group facilitation
Lecturing
Team development
Management and leadership of educational change
Quality assurance, enhancement and evaluation

Overall satisfaction with the programmes described in the papers analysed was high, with participants reporting improvements in their own teaching behaviours which were also picked up by students. Other reported changes included greater educational involvement and the development of collegial networks. However, the evidence that faculty development makes a difference to outcomes is somewhat thin on the ground. A review by the Academy of Medical Educators (2009b) found that, despite some low level evidence cited elsewhere (Kilminster et al, 2007), no high quality controlled trials or systematic reviews could be found that robustly demonstrated a causal link between trainer development programmes and enhancements in trainee progress or patient outcomes. That is not to say that there is no benefit, but the research has yet be done.

Careers in medical education

From the time of Hippocrates, medical education was viewed as something essential to the very nature of being a doctor, but also perhaps as something exercised on an ad hoc and amateur basis by any doctor, to any willing student. Now, throughout undergraduate and postgraduate medicine there are many opportunities for doctors to engage in increasingly well-defined educational roles. Students and trainees participate in teaching and there are many university and health service departments and other organizations devoted to medical education.

For clinical teachers, challenges remain about the time allocated to undertake these activities and the extent to which medical education is recognized and valued within service institutions. Clinical excellence awards recognize teaching and training but only as a small component of the application, and arguments about the appropriate time required in consultant job plans (and where to find it from) continue to rage. And so, to a frustrating extent, we continue, at least for the moment, to fall back on the goodwill of colleagues, their professional values and Hippocratic obligations.

Some of the more common and well-defined roles in medical education found in the hospital setting are described here:

Undergraduate

Clinical teachers

Although nomenclature varies between different medical schools and service providers, all medical schools have a large number of clinical teachers who are required to provide teaching for students at all stages of the programme in their speciality. Some teachers will have honorary medical school appointments (e.g. senior lecturer or professor) whereas others may simply have one or two sessions allocated to teaching and assessing students funded through the Service Increment for Teaching but will not have an academic post.

Educational coordination and management

A smaller number of posts exist in which clinicians take on a wider range of responsibilities and activities on behalf of a medical school. These are usually joint appointments between the school and the NHS employer. In addition to leading clinical departments, other typical cross-programme roles include leadership or coordination of years or phases, clinical teaching and clinical assessment. These roles involve participation in curriculum committees, curriculum review and development, educational research and other medical school activities.

Academic training posts

Increasingly, special posts are being funded by schools (and/or deaneries) such as academic teaching fellows (these may be in certain specialities or more broadly) which provide opportunities for continuing clinical training, educational research and teaching students or trainees while undertaking an educational development programme such as a postgraduate certificate in medical or clinical education.

Postgraduate

Postgraduate educational supervisor

An educational supervisor is responsible for the overall supervision and management of a trainee's educational progress during a training placement or series of placements. The educational supervisor is responsible for the trainee's educational agreement and for reporting on trainee progress to the postgraduate deanery.

Postgraduate clinical supervisor

A clinical supervisor is responsible for overseeing a specified trainee's clinical work and providing constructive feedback during a training placement. Sometimes the role is merged with the educational supervisor in which case the 'baton' of educational supervision is handed on from one placement to the next.

Training programme director

The training programme director is responsible for the orchestration of training placements and programmes for postgraduate trainees.

Director of medical education

The director of medical education is responsible for maintaining and developing the profile of education within a trust and ensuring the delivery of the deanery educational contract. He/she is usually a trust employee but has a close professional relationship with the deanery to ensure quality control of programmes, develop and deliver the wider multi-professional educational agenda and for supporting and developing tutors as educators.

Postgraduate dean

Postgraduate deans commission and manage the delivery of postgraduate education for all doctors and dentists in training. They ensure that training opportunities are available to meet future workforce needs and are responsible for recruitment to training placements and programmes. Through a network of associate deans, directors and specialty schools, postgraduate deans also manage a process of quality assurance against standards for training set by the Postgraduate Medical Education and Training Board. Deans and deaneries also play an important role in supporting the continuing professional development of a number of professional groups (e.g. GPs, staff and associate specialists, dentists).

Continuing professional development

College tutor

Before Modernising Medical Careers (Department of Health, 2003) and the establishment in deaneries of specialty schools, college tutors played a central role in the quality monitoring of training placements and the oversight of the training of junior hospital doctors. This is now not universally the case, and the college tutor role has become less easy to define. The level of involvement in local education varies from trust to trust and across specialties but college tutors continue to be the professional representative at the level of the local organization.

Medical director

Ensuring consultant participation in continuing professional development is ultimately the responsibility of the medical directors of NHS trusts through the appraisal process and a network of appraisal leads. Depending on the college and the individual relationships at local level, encouragement and monitoring of continuing professional development in some instances has been devolved to tutors.

In addition the roles listed, numerous opportunities are also available for those with an interest in medical education ranging from acting as a facilitator in a local simulation centre, becoming an examiner for either a medical school or a Royal College and engaging in educational research.

The future for medical educators

The trends outlined above are only likely to continue and as indicated in Chapter 1, training the trainers is no longer an optional extra.With the advent of revalidation, educational roles and responsibilities are likely to become further and more clearly defined.

In the university sector, medical education is now regarded as a speciality in its own right and the worldwide shortage of clinical academics has stimulated a new focus on recruiting and retaining clinicians who will take a lead in medical education. *Tomorrow's Doctors* (GMC, 2009) suggests that medical students should be trained in basic teaching skills and have the opportunity to teach others. Although this poses the challenge of fitting yet another topic into crowded undergraduate curricula, it also means that, over time, more doctors will be formally trained to teach and they will not acquire these skills opportunistically or serendipitously. Junior doctors too are now being recruited as educators with academic training paths identified at both foundation and specialty levels. For example some academic clinical fellowships are specifically structured around medical education (National Institute for Health Research, 2010). Departments of medical and clinical education provide a focus for academic activities, including research and professional development programmes. There will therefore be increasing opportunities for medical students and doctors in training to take on roles in medical education, with the possible future development of medical education as a defined clinical sub-specialty.

Although all doctors will emerge from medical schools with basic teaching skills, in future not everyone will be required to teach and train, and those that do so will have to demonstrate that they have the ability to do so. The introduction of professional standards means that those who wish to make a career in teaching will be able to obtain recognition and career pathways in medical education will become more clearly defined and appropriately remunerated. Already we are starting to see full-time appointments made in large trusts to Director of Medical Education positions.

As novel patient pathways and integrated services continue to break down the historical boundaries between professional groups, we will also see more need for interprofessional educators who can work with, teach and assess multiprofessional groups. Meeting the needs of medical educators will place more emphasis on being able to provide support for clinicians to identify their educational development needs, introducing flexible training and development programmes that fit around busy clinical commitments and providing pathways and programmes for career advancement in medical education by organizations, specialties and professional bodies. This will require effective, collaborative and informed educational leadership. Organizations and individuals will need to work closely together in order to provide seamless faculty and professional development, training and career opportunities, reward and recognize effort and aspiration and ensure that the students and trainees of tomorrow receive the highest quality education and training.

KEY POINTS

- Doctors who teach students and trainees are increasingly required to be able to demonstrate their teaching expertise.
- Professional development activities help clinicians to improve their teaching.
- Professional standards for medical educators enable individual clinicians and organizations to benchmark teaching practice and gain recognition.
- A wide range of professional development opportunities in medical education exist for students, trainees and qualified doctors.
- An increasing number of roles in medical education are available for doctors who want to be involved in education and training.

References

Academy of Medical Educators (2009a) *Professional Standards Framework*. Academy of Medical Educators, London

Academy of Medical Educators (2009b) *Educational supervisors in secondary care Stage 1 report*. Academy of Medical Educators, London (www.medicaleducators.org/resources. asp accessed 13 February 2010)

Darzi A (2008) *A High Quality Workforce: NHS Next Stage Review*. Department of Health, London

Department of Health (2003) *Modernising Medical Careers*. Department of Health, London

Flexner A (1910) *Medical Education in the United States and Canada: A Report to the Carnegie Foundation for the Advancement of Teaching*. Carnegie Foundation for the Advancement of Teaching, New York

General Medical Council (2009) *Tomorrows Doctors*. GMC, London

Higher Education Academy (2006) *The UK Professional Standards Framework for teaching and supporting learning in higher education*. Higher Education Academy, York (www. heacademy.ac.uk/ourwork/policy/framework accessed 10 January 2010)

Kilminster S, Cottrell D, Grant J, Jolly B (2007) AMEE Guide No. 27: Effective educational and clinical supervision. *Med Teach* **29**: 2–19

London Deanery (2009) *Professional Development Framework for Supervisors*. London Deanery, London (http://faculty.londondeanery.ac.uk/professional-development-framework-for-supervisors accessed 10 January 2010)

McKimm J, Swanwick T (2010) Educational leadership. In: Swanwick T, McKimm J, eds. *ABC of Clinical Leadership*. Wiley Blackwell, London

National Institute for Health Research (2010) NIHR Integrated Academic Training. NIHR, London (www.nihrtcc.nhs.uk/intetacatrain/ accessed 12 January 2010)

Postgraduate Medical Education and Training Board (2008) *Educating Tomorrows Doctors - Future models of medical training; medical workforce shape and trainee expectations*. PMETB, London

Steinert Y, Mann K, Centeno A, Dolmans D, Spencer J, Gelula M, Prideaux D (2006) A systematic review of faculty development initiatives designed to improve teaching effectiveness in medical education. *Med Teach* **28**: 497–526

Swanwick T (2008) See one, do one, then what? Faculty development in postgraduate medical education. *Postgrad Med J* **84**(993): 339–43

Tooke J (2008) *Aspiring to excellence: Findings and recommendations of the independent inquiry into modernising medical careers*. Universities UK, London

CHAPTER 23

Assuring and enhancing educational quality

Mark Barrow and Judy McKimm

Clinical teachers need to evaluate the quality and effectiveness of their teaching. Evaluation of teaching and learning generally occurs within quality assurance frameworks that have common features. Understanding quality assurance systems and evaluation methods will help clinical teachers to improve the student learning experience.

This chapter discusses how quality assurance systems used in medical and health professions' education function within an overall quality improvement agenda and introduces the most common tools used in the evaluation of teaching and learning.

Introduction

Higher and professional education in the western world has undergone rapid change. The expansion of student numbers, widening diversity and opening access, the impact of e-learning systems that facilitate distance learning, and increasing recognition of the importance of workplace learning have led to concerns over maintaining and enhancing educational quality across a diverse sector.

Addressing such concerns has led all establishments with educational missions, from schools to universities as well as institutions such as Medical Royal Colleges and postgraduate deaneries, to place greater emphasis on demonstrating:

- Quality improvement
- Accountability for spending public money
- Transparency of processes involving admissions, teaching and assessment
- The specification and achievement of competencies and outcomes
- Early identification and remediation of 'failing' students or practitioners.

The 'quality agenda' in clinical education has recently seen movement on a number of fronts towards explicit standard-setting, evidence-based education, metrics and indicators to measure continuous improvement, and the establishment of structures and processes that enable self-governance and monitoring. The quality agenda therefore impacts on all aspects of education at all levels from funding and regulatory bodies, through to educational providers and ultimately to teachers and learners.

What is quality?

'Quality' has been described in various ways in industry and in other areas such as higher education. A useful description is that provided in *Figure 23.1*).

Quality assurance refers to the policies, processes and actions through which quality is maintained, developed, monitored and demonstrated (McKimm, 2009). The way in which quality is perceived has implications both for the way in which systems are set up and how quality is measured, including defining standards, performance criteria or learning outcomes.

Figure 23.1. Defining quality.
From Harvey and Green (1993).

As **exceptional or excellent** — quality is seen as something special or distinctive, demonstrating the highest academic standards or conversely, meeting a threshold standard

As **perfection** — here quality represents consistent or flawless outcomes. This 'democratises' the notion of quality, suggesting that if consistency can be achieved then quality can be attained by all

As **fitness for purpose** — in terms of fulfilling requirements or needs. In education, this view is usually based on the ability of an institution to fulfil its mission or of a programme to fulfil its aims. Quality here relates to the extent to which a product or service fits its purpose

As **value for money** — funding bodies and students increasingly expect a value for money approach. They want to know that the same outcome could not be achieved at a lower cost or that it is not possible to achieve a better outcome at the same cost

As **transformation or enhancement** — this view sees quality in terms of change from one state to another. In education, transformation refers to both the enhancement (value-added) and empowerment of students

Evaluation

A key element of quality assurance in education is evaluation (*see Figure 11.2 on page 105*).

Ramsden (1992) describes evaluation as: 'a way of understanding the effects of our teaching on students' learning. It implies collecting information about our work, interpreting the information and making judgements about which actions we should take to improve practice ... evaluation is an analytical process that is critical to good teaching'.

Kirkpatrick (1994) suggests that evaluation should be carried out at four levels: reaction (or satisfaction) with the learning process, learning (of knowledge and skills), behaviour or capability to perform skills, and results, impact, outcomes or transfer of learning to the workplace. Organizations are usually good at gathering information from and about students and programmes at the lower levels of evaluation but tend to be much less effective in using it to enhance the quality of their education provision.

Learners also commonly complain that nothing seems to change as a result of their feedback. This leads students to become resistant to exercises designed to elicit feedback, providing misleading data or refusing to participate. Teachers need to demonstrate and explain what is going to change as a result and also what is not going to change.

The quality assurance cycle

One of the outcomes of the quality movement has been the development of a specialized bureaucracy to ensure smooth operation of (often complex) quality systems including apparatuses for audit and accountability. Quality assurance systems at system, organizational or individual level typically operate within a cycle (*Figure 23.2*).

Quality assurance agencies expect staff at all levels in institutions (including classroom and clinical teachers) to gather data that allow them to demonstrate these steps and the manner in which each step affects and feeds into the next.

Key features of the quality assurance process

Regardless of the agency or the object of scrutiny, there is a reasonably common approach to reviews, be they audit, approval or accreditation. The key features of quality assurance include:

- Self evaluation – usually through a review report in which the institution provides a self-assessment of its activities relating to the scope of the review
- External expert review conducted by an autonomous agency – usually involving documentary scrutiny and a visit by reviewers to the institution
- The public report – with commentary and recommendations
- Benchmarking – periodic reviews by the agency across the sector to identify common themes and issues.

While most review and evaluation systems are developed on the basis of promoting ongoing improvement, review systems need to be robust enough to stop under-performing institutions, subjects or programmes from receiving monies from governments or other funders or from taking students.

Systems of quality assurance in medical education

Health professions' education occurs in a range of contexts, carried out by a variety of institutions and professional bodies. The locus of control in these areas depends on whether the health professional is a student, trainee or independent practitioner. Although each healthcare profession has its own unique set of educational structures and processes, there are similarities across the disciplines.

Figure 23.2. The quality assurance cycle.

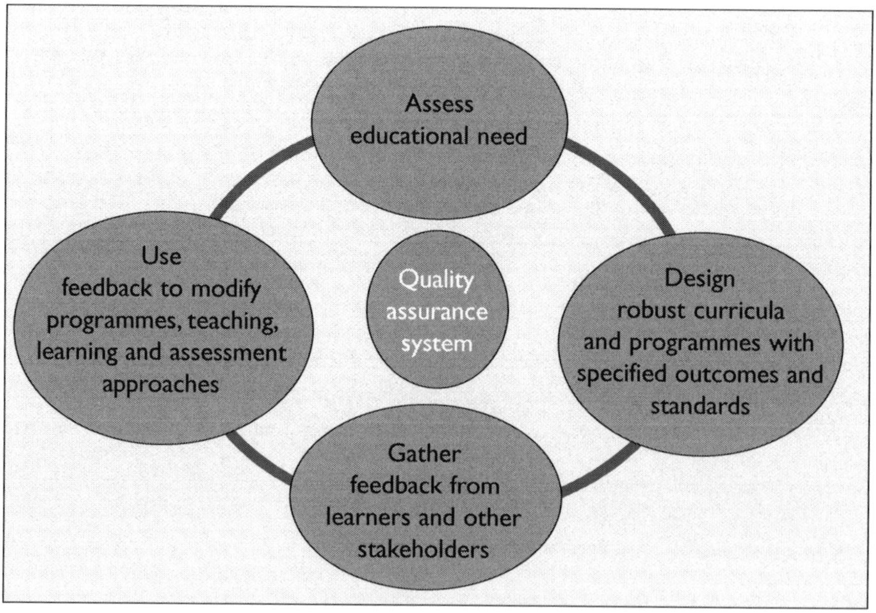

The undergraduate context

Students preparing for professional registration are generally enrolled in university programmes which, although relying on practicing clinicians for much of the teaching, remain under the control of universities and through them the agencies that have a mandate for audit. These agencies are primarily concerned with assuring governments that taxpayers are getting value for money and that graduates are fit for purpose.

In the UK, undergraduate medical education is funded by the Higher Education Funding Councils and the Department of Health (to support clinical placements). Quality assurance is carried out by the Quality Assurance Agency and by the Department of Health through monitoring of funding streams that support clinical education. The Quality Assurance Agency is an independent body working across all higher education provision under contract from the Higher Education Funding Councils.

Professional and statutory bodies also have a role in the approval and accreditation of undergraduate programmes offered by universities to assure fitness for purpose of graduates. The General Medical Council manages this through the Quality Assurance of Basic Medical Education (QABME) process (General Medical Council, 2009). These mechanisms assure professional bodies that programmes meet defined 'threshold' standards in terms of curriculum outcomes and delivery methods and that the provider institution has resources, systems and governance arrangements to ensure appropriate delivery of the approved programme. Initial approval and accreditation is followed up with a cycle of reviews and audits.

The postgraduate context

In the UK, the Department of Health is responsible for specifying the curriculum for foundation trainees and medical Royal Colleges are responsible for determining the curricula, carrying out assessments for trainees in various specialities, revalidation and professional development. The responsibility for ensuring that the educational experience of trainees meets quality standards falls to the General Medical Council (which took on this responsibility when the Postgraduate Medical Education and Training Board merged with the General Medical Council in April 2010). Regional deaneries carry out quality monitoring and evaluation of educational organizations in their area.

Continuing professional development and revalidation

In terms of continuing professional development and revalidation, quality assurance processes are influenced by a number of policy shifts. These include further formalizing revalidation, recertification and licensing (quality assured by the General Medical Council and Royal Colleges), a shift towards specification of competencies at all levels, a greater emphasis on educational and clinical supervision and formalizing staff and educational development (See Chapter 22). In response to these shifts, new professional standards frameworks for teachers and supervisors are being introduced, adding another layer to the quality assurance processes (Postgraduate Medical Education and Training Board, 2008; Academy of Medical Educators, 2009).

The role of the clinical teacher

Although many organizations have central or departmental quality units or groups with a responsibility for ensuring that data are gathered, reports are submitted and reviews are carried out, the individual teacher plays a key role in assuring and improving quality. The professionalization of medical education places increasing scrutiny on all teachers and raises expectation about them. Review exercises are based on an expectation that individual teachers build quality assurance and evaluation processes into their own teaching practice. In particular they are concerned with the extent to which learning outcomes are aligned with teaching and learning methods, assessment methods and evaluation (Biggs, 1996), and the ways in which teachers act on misalignment in a continual review cycle (see *Figure 11.2 on page 105*).

Learners are at the heart of any educational review cycle. Gathering information about learners – their levels of satisfaction, engagement in learning and achievement of agreed learning outcomes or objectives – is the foundation of all quality systems. These data provide the best information upon which a clinical teacher might base his or her reflections on the need for and means of improving the alignment of outcomes, methods and assessment.

A good teacher needs to be in a position to gather information and to respond to it. In addition he/she needs to maintain the sort of records that will allow him/her to assure organizations and external agencies that he/she is gathering robust information and that the information is used to constantly scrutinize his/her assumptions about student learning.

Gathering and using feedback

One of the key elements of any quality assurance system is ensuring that the data are collated efficiently into a form which can be analysed and that they are presented appropriately. In order to achieve this we need to consider the most appropriate sorts of data.

Hounsell (2009) suggests that data should be gathered from a range of sources including:

- Feedback from students
- Self-generated feedback, e.g. gathered from audio or video observation
- Feedback from colleagues, e.g. peer evaluation
- Incidental feedback, e.g. attendance patterns, take up of options, attentiveness.

Gathering evaluative data from students plays an important role in tracking student satisfaction and engagement over time and can be effective at course, programme and institutional level. The majority of clinical teachers will be involved in formally evaluating learning and constantly gauge the progress learners are making and adjust their approaches to enhance this. For example, skillfully asking questions of learners to ascertain how much they have learned or areas of confusion gives the teacher the data he or she needs to alter approaches to teaching or lesson content (See Chapter 7). This reflective approach is a hallmark of excellent teaching which does not lend itself to formal systematization other than through peer review and reflective portfolios maintained for professional development purposes.

In addition, other routinely held institutional data on assessment performance, admissions information or graduate employment may provide useful feedback on the quality and relevance of education.

The quality assurance 'tool' most commonly used at classroom level is the student feedback questionnaire, this typically considers either student satisfaction or learner engagement with the learning process. Satisfaction surveys are typically designed to gather data from learners about courses or teachers. Questionnaires designed to gather both quantitative and qualitative data tend to be the most common method of gathering this information. Student or trainee satisfaction data provides information to teachers and institutions about the way students feel about the learning processes in which they are participating. Such systems may be applied nationally. In the UK, the National Student Survey gathers information about all students in higher education and the Postgraduate Medical Education and Training Board carries out national training surveys of all medical trainees.

Satisfaction feedback is often criticized by those who believe that it emphasizes the wrong things if learning is the goal: a learner who is 'satisfied' or 'happy' still may not be learning. Student engagement questionnaires aim to ascertain the extent to which learning activities stimulate students to become engaged in educationally purposeful activities. Much work has been done by international agencies and consortia in distilling information. For example surveys developed in the US (the National Survey of Student Engagement – www.nsse.iub.edu) and Australasia (the Australasian Survey of Student Engagement – http://ausse.acer.edu.au/) provide information about the level of student engagement prompted by teaching.

A frequent criticism of feedback questionnaires is that they tend, because of the complexity of their design and administration, to be used at the end of the course in a form of 'summative' evaluation. Teachers cannot use the data to modify their approach to teaching or the emphasis of the course to benefit the learners directly, instead the benefit tends to be for future learners. Students can become disenchanted with such systems as it is very hard to demonstrate that their feedback results in improvements. Also, because many of the data gathered from these exercises are quantitative, relatively large sample sizes are required to draw meaningful conclusions. For a reflective educator working with small cohorts of learners or seeking to make improvements on a day-to-day basis, this type of survey has reduced efficacy.

Many other techniques can be used to systematically gather learner feedback so as to make timely changes to teaching. Examples include small group instructional diagnosis (a facilitated small group discussion to provide feedback from learners to the teacher; Floren, 2002) and the 'one-minute paper' (Angelo and Cross, 1993) which can provide teachers with timely post-session information about what is working or not working for students.

Conclusions

Assuring and maintaining quality in clinical education is a complex process involving multiple agencies, institutions and individuals. Policy and practice agendas in education and health emphasize the need for continuous monitoring, review and evaluation of all processes from management systems through to day to day teaching activities. Clinical teachers may be involved in a range of data gathering and evaluation activities and play a central role in gathering and using feedback from learners, peers and others to improve their teaching. The reflective teacher also uses opportunities for self-reflection and review to improve the quality of learning and teaching.

> # KEY POINTS
>
> *   Quality assurance and evaluation activities are key to improving learning and teaching
> *   Student feedback is central to improving quality, but is not the only method or indicator
> *   Teachers can use a mix of formal survey questionnaires and informal feedback to improve teaching
> *   Evaluation is part of the 'plan – do – reflect – review' cycle of the reflective practitioner

References

Academy of Medical Educators (2009) *Professional Standards Framework*. Academy of Medical Educators, London

Angelo TA, Cross KP (1993) *Classroom Assessment Techniques: A Handbook for College Teachers*. 2nd edn. Jossey-Bass, San Francisco, CA

Biggs J (1996) Enhancing learning through constructive alignment. *Higher Education* **32**: 347–64

Floren G (2002) Evaluating Teaching through SGID. www.miracosta.edu/home/gfloren/ sgid.htm (accessed 24 March 2010)

General Medical Council (2009) *Overview of the QABME programme*. General Medical Council, London (www.gmc-uk.org/education/undergraduate/qabme_programme.asp accessed 17 March 2010)

Harvey L, Green D (1993) Defining quality. *Assessment and Evaluation in Higher Education* **18**(1): 9–34

Hounsell D (2009) Evaluating courses and teaching. In: Fry H, Ketteridge S, Marshall S, eds. *A handbook for teaching and learning in higher education: enhancing academic practice*. 3rd edn. Routledge, London: 198–211

Kirkpatrick DL (1994) *Evaluating Training Programs*. Berrett-Koehler Publishers, Inc, San Francisco

London Deanery (2008) The educational paradigm. www.faculty.londondeanery.ac.uk/e-learning/setting-learning-objectives/the-educational-paradigm (accessed 15 May 2009)

McKimm J (2009) Quality, standards and enhancement. In: Fry H, Ketteridge S, Marshall S, eds. *A handbook for teaching and learning in higher education: enhancing academic practice*. 3rd edn. Routledge, London: 186–97

Postgraduate Medical Education and Training Board (2008) *Educating Tomorrows Doctors - Future models of medical training; medical workforce shape and trainee expectations*. Postgraduate Medical Education and Training Board, London

Quality Assurance Agency (2002) *Subject Benchmark Statements: Academic Standards, Medicine*. Quality Assurance Agency, Gloucester (www.qaa.ac.uk/academicinfrastructure/benchmark/honours/medicine.asp accessed 26 February 2010)

Ramsden P (1992) *Learning to Teach in Higher Education*. 2nd edn. Routledge, London

Index

Academy of Medical Educators
    Professional Standards
    Framework 221
accountability 220
action research 215
active learning 77
active listening 160
affective domain 24
aims 17, 36
appraisal 53, 175
  active listening 160
  benefits 154
  communication cycle 157–8
  defined 153–4
  environment 156–7
  feedback 157
  interview 157–8
  managing 153–62
  NHS scheme 155
  objectives as output from 160–1
  preparation for 156
  questioning 159–60
  self-assessment 158–9
assessment
  interprofessional learning 119
  long and short cases 146
  structured 145–51
  workplace-based *see* workplace-based
    assessment
assessment methods 38
attitudinal objectives 24
audit 14

Bloom's taxonomy of objectives 20–1
blueprinting 148

career decision making 167–8
career exploration 166–7
career planning 169–70
career planning workshops 165
careers 55
careers support 163–70
  career decision making 167–8
  career exploration 166–7
  framework 164
  interview preparation 168–9
  need for 163
  plan implementation 168
  providers of 164
  self-assessment 164–5
  unrealistic plans 169
case study 215
case-based discussion 67
challenges for teachers 222
clinical teachers, role of 7–8
clinical teaching 117–18
coaching 53, 175–6
collaboration 114
communities of practice 64, 116
competencies 18, 35–6
  feedback and 46
competency frameworks 3–4
confidentiality 98
consent 97
constructive alignment 119, 127–8
continuing professional
    development 155, 236
  careers 226–7
counselling 175
course design 29–40
cultural competence 197–8

curricular cycle   30
curriculum
  centralized/decentralized   31
  content   37
  design   29–40
  design models   33
  evaluation   39
  formal   29
  hidden   29
  implementing   38
  integrated   35
  key elements   36–8
  monitoring   39
  objectives model   32
  pre-clinical/clinical models   34
  process model   32–3
  spiral   33
  strategies and approaches   31–3

deliberate practice   138–9
difficult trainees   191–2
direct observation of procedural
      skills   108, 189
disability   195–6
discrimination
  anti-discriminatory framework   199–
      200
  case scenarios   203–4
  challenging behaviour   204
  institutional   198
  key legal principles   200–1
  legal issues   199–200
  teaching context   203
diversity   195–205
  defined   196
  importance of   196–7
  valuing   197
DOPS see direct observation of
      procedural skills

e-assessment   123
e-learning   123–30
  contact between teacher and
      pupil   125
  content   126
  defined   123–4

development template   129
  models of   124–8
  planning and implementing   128–9
  process   126
equality   195–205
  defined   195
  importance of   196–7
  see also discrimination
e-teaching   123
ethical issues   97–8
ethnography   215
evidence   107–9
  educational research   207–8
expert patients   95–6

feedback   41–9
  absence of   138
  appraisal   157
  barriers to   44–5
  formal   47–8
  giving   43–4
  informal   45–6
  models of   44
  negative   45
  patients   64
  quality assurance   237–8
  receiving   48
  role of   41
  workplace-based assessment   109
focus groups   215
formal assessment tools   14
forming   81

gender   195–6
General Medical Council, Good
      Medical Practice   1–2
graduate entry   34
group size and dynamics   80–2

harassment   201
horizontal learning   65–6
human rights   202–3

integrated teaching   104–5
  simulation   138
interprofessional education   114

interprofessional learning   113–121
  assessment   119
  challenges   119–20
  clinical teaching   117–18
  communities of practice   116
  defined   113–14
  drivers for   115
  principles of   115–16
  role of teacher   118
invitational workplaces   64

job planning   175
Johari window   9

knowledge objectives   23
knowledge paradigms   208
Kolb's experiential learning cycle   11,
    42–3, 62

labelling   63
learner-centred learning   86
learning methods   37
learning needs
  assessing   7–15
  Johari window   9
  teacher assessment of   12
  techniques   12–13
learning objectives *see* objectives
learning on ward rounds   208–11
learning process, feedback and   42
learning resources   38
learning theory   117
learning through participation   62, 65
learning through talking   66
leaving medicine   168
lectures
  aims and outcomes   72
  characteristics of   71–2
  first five minutes   75
  level of new content   74–5
  purpose of   72
  structure   72–4
lecturing   69–77
  audio-visual aids   76
  defined   69
  engaging the audience   76

from notes   76
  handouts   76
  practising   75
  reasons for   69–70
lesson planning   24–5
lifelong learning   169

manikins   135, 139
medical education   3
  careers   224–7
  future   227–8
  trends   31
medical education research   207–17
  data   216
  designing   213–16
  dimensions of research quality   212
  fitness for purpose   209, 212
  qualitative studies   213–14
  qualitative vs. quantitative   208–9
  sampling methods   214–15
mentoring   52–3, 173–83
  benefits   176–7
  defined   173–4
  ineffective   182–3
  mentees   180
  principles   179–80
  questions   181–2
  scheme   178–9
  skills needed   179–80
  successful   177–9
  trainees in difficulty   192–3
  traps   182
  types of   179
  typical topics   177
Miller's pyramid   21–2, 103–4
mini-clinical evaluation exercise (mini-
    CEX)   108, 189
multiprofessional education   114

norming   81

objective structured clinical
    examinations   145–51
  blueprinting   148–9
  characteristics of   147
  defined   146

educational impact 147–8
examiners 150
global ratings vs. checklist
    scores 150
real patients 150
reliability of 147
simulated patients 149
station development 148–9
validity of 147
objectives 17, 160–1
attitudinal 24
domains 22
knowledge 23
setting 17–27
skills 23–4
writing 22–4
OSCEs see objective structured clinical
    examinations
outcomes 18, 36
hierarchies of 18–19
pitfalls 25–7
writing 22–4

patient involvement 91–100
benefit to patients 93
choice of patients 92–6
defined 91–2
disadvantages 92
ethical issues 97–8
expert patients 95–6
location 94
opportunities 98–9
patients' views 96–7
real patients 95
reasons for 92
video and audio 96
patients, simulation 133–42
patronage 174
performing 82
personal development plans 14
plan, do, reflect, review cycle 11
planning 11
portfolios 14–15, 109–10
positive action 201
postgraduate teaching 225–6

prejudice 201
problem-based learning 35
process-driven model 20
professional competence 10
professional conversations 12–13
professional development
competency model 9
frameworks 220–2
learning objectives and 20
medical educators 219–28
role of feedback 46
types of 223–4
psychometric testing 165
public duties 200, 202
pursuit of excellence 220

quality assurance 110–11, 231–9
continuing professional
    development 236
cycle 233–4
evaluation 233
feedback 237–8
postgraduate teaching 235
role of teachers 236
systems 234–5
undergraduate teaching 235
quality, defined 232

race 195–6
regulation 2
religion 195–6
revalidation 2, 236
ROADS 167
rule of threes 74

self-assessment 158–9
seven principles 124–5
sexuality 195–6
significant event analysis 13
simulation 133–42
in assessment 149–50
benefits of 135
best practice 137
future of 141–2
learning and 136–7

limitations   140–1
in practice   139–40
reasons for   134
types of   135–6
skills   2–4
skills objectives   23–4
small group teaching   79–89
closing the session   88–9
handling problems   88
planning and preparation   83–5
question strategies   87–8
role of teacher   80–1
room layout   84–5
session types   82–3
starting the session   85
strategies   85–6
structuring   82
small groups, defined   79
SMART   22, 161
social class   195–6
social identity   196
sociocultural learning theories   62–3
standardized assessments   104–5
storming   82
stress   191–2
supervision   3, 51–9, 175
benefits of   53
care   57
cases   54
caution   57
clinical   52
complexity   57
constraints   55–6
contexts   54, 57
conversations   56
creativity   57
curiosity   56
domains of   51
educational   52
good practice   53
power and   55
process   58
seven Cs   56–7
useful questions   58–9
supporting students   7
systematic review   215

TAPUPAS model   212
teachers, teaching   1–2
teaching, group sizes
teaching methods   37
teamworking   114
technology   124, 134, 142
therapy   174
thinking aloud   66
threshold competence   36
trainee talk   66–7
trainees in difficulty   185–193
career development issues   191
diagnosing   185–6
difficult trainees   191–2
health issues   190
interventions   188–9
learning environment   188
mentoring   192–3
personal issues   190–1
signs of   186–7
stress   191–2
supporting   187–91
training, roles and responsibilities   186
Tuckman's model of group process   81
tutor-centred learning   86

undergraduate teaching   224–5
underperforming doctors   155
uni-professional learning   114

victimisation   201

Web 2.0   126–7
workplace-based assessment   103–11
analysis of performance data   109
blueprinted   106
competency-based   106
defined   103–4
developmental   106–7
discussion of clinical cases   108
evidence   107–9
feedback   109
observation   108
portfolios   109–10
quality assurance   110–11
usefulness   104–5

workplace-based learning 61–7
  challenges 61–2
  opportunities 63

World Health Organization 113